W9-BYB-532

Sarcoidosis

Resource Guide and Directory

A Medical Mystery Uncovered,
Facts, Information and Helplines

By

Sandra Conroy

First Edition

PC Publications, Piscataway, New Jersey

Sarcoidosis

Resource Guide and Directory

By Sandra Conroy

Published by:

 PC Publications
P.O. Box 1593
Piscataway,N.J. 08855-1593

Library of Congress Catalog Card Number: 91-91267
Conroy, Sandra E.
Sarcoidosis Resource Guide and Directory
ISBN 0-9631222-5-8 $19.95 Softcover

Table of Contents

Part 1

Chapter I

Chapter II

Chapter III

Chapter IV

Part 2

Directories

Part 3

Appendix A

Appendix B

Appendix C

About The Author

I have been living with Sarcoidosis for eight years. After much soul searching and learning about the disease, I have been able to reconstruct some of my earlier symptoms. At the time, however, I had no knowledge of the existence of Sarcoidosis, much less its symptoms.

In the winter of 1978, I was living in Yonkers, N.Y. with my husband Robert, and our two sons, Andre and Michael. I worked on Wall Street, commuting to New York City on the railroad. I was manager of a Data Processing Department, which often required a ten to twelve hour work day, plus a two hour commute each way. It was my husband's custom to meet me at the train. While on my way home one night, I began to feel a pricking sensation (like needles and pins) on the side of my face. After a minute or two, the sensation went away. At the time, I attributed the feeling to being overtired and put it out of my mind. I now recall that I had experienced that same type of sensation several times during that year.

Robert and I always planned special family activities for our children. The summer of 1979 is frozen in my memory. We were at Bear Mountain in upstate New York with our children and friends. I had been roller skating and decided to stop and go back to the picnic area. While walking through the woods, I suddenly could not lift my left leg. I managed to get back to the picnic area by dragging my left leg. Once I reached the picnic area, I sat down and just as quickly as it appeared, the numbness went away. Several weeks later, I experienced the same type of episode. This time, we were at an amusement park. Both times the symptoms seemed to last about ten minutes.

Being able to wear high heel shoes everyday, and suffering no more symptoms, I soon forgot all about the episodes. I soon discovered that on weekends, when I would take off the heels and put on flat shoes or sneakers, I would have recurring episodes of my leg dragging.

Finally, I went into the hospital for tests. Naturally all of my tests were negative. The doctors had no answer, and so for the next two years I wore high heel shoes and was able to manage. However, I knew something was wrong. I developed a dry cough during the late summer of 1983. While at work, I had a coughing spell, which caused me to start bleeding through my nose. I started to run a temperature, and was hospitalized for six weeks with a diagnosis of pneumonia. After being released from the hospital, I began having a low grade fever, which would start in the late afternoon or early evening. I also had night sweats and would have to get up and change my nightgown three or four times nightly. In addition, my left leg became inflamed and I had severe knee pain. I also noticed dark blotches around my left ankle and neck, and my eyes became swollen, blurring my vision.

By this time, we had moved to New Jersey and my neighbor recommended that I see her doctor. After taking my case history, the doctor felt that I might have Sarcoidosis. For further testing, he sent me to the Hospital at the University of Pennsylvania.

Finally, in 1984, it was discovered that I indeed had Sarcoidosis. An ophthalmologist treated my eyes, and for one year I had to use a solution called Tears. Gradually the blotches, the inflammation, and fever disappeared. However, my left leg still continued to drag, and I began having problems with my foot as well. I developed what is called footdrop.

By the spring of 1985, my leg began dragging more frequently; I found that I had trouble lifting at all. Stairs became impossible. I had to climb one step at a time using my right leg. In September of that year, I was again admitted to the hospital at the University of Pennsylvania. Again, I went through a barrage of testing. Once again doctors were baffled. My symptoms and clinical studies did not add up to a clear, concise diagnosis.

I was told that I had Sarcoidosis, possible Multiple Sclerosis, and nerve damage that I had suffered from a previous accident. Because of my inability to lift my leg and the footdrop, I was fitted for a leg brace. I also started to use a cane.

I had two operations and spent the next five years going to physical therapy. During this time, everyone I encountered knew nothing about Sarcoidosis or of its existence. I felt isolated, and began to wonder, if I was the only one on this planet with this disease.

Not one to give up or wallow in self pity, I was determined to make the best of things. I joined a Multiple Sclerosis support group. I learned that support groups are important for people with a chronic illness.

Finally in 1990, I discovered that there was a Sarcoidosis Foundation and a support group in Newark, New Jersey. For the first time, I met people that could really understand what I was going through, for they too shared the same physical symptoms and had pondered the same unanswered questions I had.

I often reflect on my past experiences: Yes,
Having a chronic disease is difficult.

--Dealing with a disability is difficult.

--Having a disease and not being able to get answers
is difficult.

--Having symptoms that have not been identified or
recognized as being consistent with the disease
is difficult.

--Not being able to find support from others afflicted
with this disease is difficult.

--Not being able to find a physician who has an
association with the disease is difficult.

--To seek information from your local library, and to
find not one book on Sarcoidosis is not only difficult,
its very frustrating.

It is my hope that, through this book, I will help you to
avoid some of the difficulties and frustrations I faced, and
you will be able to find some of the answers, and the
support that you need.

Sandra Conroy

Acknowledgment

Together we will make a difference, through education, and commitment. This book has been a collaborative effort. Thanks to the many contributions and talent of others, we are able to present to you the Sarcoidosis Resource Guide and Directory.

National Sarcoidosis Family Aid and Research
Geneva Ausley contribution toward research
Gracie Davis - Sarcoidosis
Self-Help Clearing House
Edward Madara - Starting a Self-Help Group
National Multiple Sclerosis Society
Robert Enteen - Social Security Disability
National Institute of Health - J. Sri Ram,Ph.D.
Nanette Alexander-Thomas, M.D. - Sarcoid Arthritis
Luther Clark, M.D. - Sarcoidosis and the Heart
Steven Faigenbaum, M.D. - Sarcoidosis and the Eye
Andrew Freedman, M.D. - Sarcoidosis and the Patient
Thomas Scott, M.D. - Neurosarcoidosis
Editors: Barbara Ames and Vikki Noble
Illustrators: Tom Betz, Kristi Bristol, Robert Conroy, and Renee Marzano. Special thanks to Della Emanuel, D'Entress Ratcliff, Dolores O'Leary, and Matthew Robinson for sharing their experiences with us. And a very special thanks to Barbara Ames, Vikki Noble and Laura Von Frolio, for their contributions, their support and their encouragement.

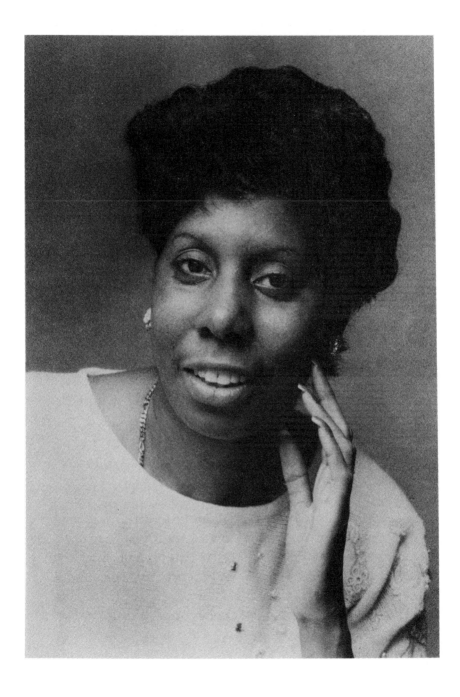

Warning--Disclaimer

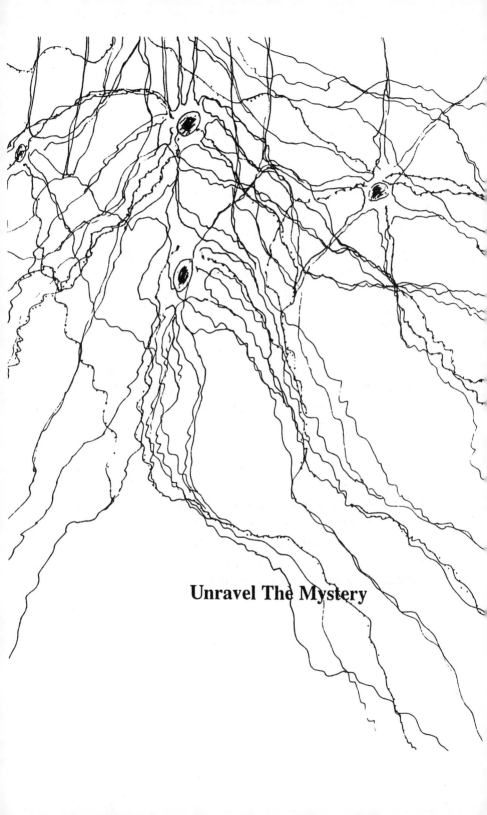

Unravel The Mystery

SARCOIDOSIS

Sarcoidosis from the Greek words "sark" and "oid", meaning "flesh-like", is an inflammatory disease. Most people have some difficulty in pronouncing the word, Sarcoidosis (Sar - coy - do - sis.) It is not surprising then, that there is widespread difficulty in understanding its symptoms and course. Sarcoidosis has been a mystery since it was first identified over one hundred years ago. Originally, it was known by the names of the two dermatologists who first identified it: Dr. Jonathan Hutchinson and Dr. Caesar Boeck's Disease until Dr. Boeck termed it Sarcoidosis, which describes the skin eruptions that often characterize the illness.

The first symptom identified was the skin involvement (dermatologic); but doctors soon observed and recorded symptoms involving the bones and eyes. Later, when radiological studies (X-rays) were developed, abnormalities of the mediastinum (thoracic or chest cavity) and pulmonary organs (lungs) were recognized as the major characteristics of this disease. Such discoveries made it possible to conclude that Sarcoidosis was a disease that could attack any bodily system or organ. Further studies showed that it could also be multisystemic: attacking two or more systems and/or organs simultaneously. It is an inflammatory disease: causing irritation, pain, swelling and heat to affected areas. It can be acute: rising rapidly to its greatest degree and followed by an inactive period of five (5) years or more. When chronic, it is marked by a long duration or by frequent reoccurrences.

Despite the advanced technological improvements in medicine, Sarcoidosis may still go undiagnosed in certain instances. For example, if a chest X-ray is taken, and the findings show a clear lung or chest cavity (free of any noticeable abnormalities), Sarcoidosis may not initially be suspected. In such cases, a person may undergo long periods of suffering before this disease is even suspected, even longer periods are endured before a diagnosis is made.

Abnormalities indicative of Sarcoidosis include, but are not limited to: Sinusitis; Fatigue (unexplainable tiredness or weakness); Ecchymosis (bruising to the skin); Migraines (headaches); Pericarditis or Endomyocarditis (inflammation of the heart); Angina Pectoris (pain in the center of the chest); Dyspnea (shortness of breath on exertion); Hypotension or Hypertension (low or high blood pressure); Hemorrhage, Iron Deficiency or Hemolytic Anemia (disorders of red blood cell components); Leukocystosis (high white blood cell count); Lymph Node Enlargement (growth of rounded capsule shaped masses of blood plasma and white blood cell liquids); Fibrosis (formation of scar tissue); Noncaseating Granulomas (formation of granular masses on chronically inflamed tissue); Nonproductive or Productive Cough (dry and nagging or presented with mucous and/or blood); Facial Paralysis (loss of function, feeling or the power of motion); Inflamed and/or enlarged pancreas, liver, kidney, or spleen; etc.

Reports vary on the incidence of Sarcoidosis. Most research indicates that African American women, ranging in age from twenty to forty (20 to 40), have the highest rate of prevalence and seriousness. Its occurrence, course, and history of remission differ among races. Exact figures have not been determined to date. Documentation of the locations where statistical data has been obtained and/or studies have been conducted is crucial.

Research verifies that women tend to outnumber men in seeking medical care. Nonwhites are treated in outpatient clinics at a significantly greater rate than whites. The latter has been attributed to economics and health education, combined with the demand for more physician resources. Regardless of the final ratio of figures, Sarcoidosis does not discriminate. It is more common than is publicly realized. It is not, however contagious.

Treatment is available for Sarcoidosis, but there is no established cure known. The medicine that has been proven to be most effective is Prednisone. It is a corticosteroid that is primarily used to decrease inflammatory responses. Many patients are fortunate: they go into remission (period during which the disease becomes inactive or burns out and relief from pain is gained) without it becoming necessary to take this drug. Prednisone has many potential side effects. They include possible adverse reactions to the brain and nervous system, skin, eyes, ears, nose, throat, digestive system, heart and lungs, muscles, bones, joints, genital and urinary tracts, blood vessels, kidneys and liver. Nevertheless, Prednisone may be prescribed in order to combat the high levels of inflammation and to prevent excessive scar tissue formation.

Even with this treatment, a greater percentage of persons with Sarcoidosis suffer permanent disabilities and withstand chronic, excruciating pain, than is publicly realized and acknowledge.

It is quite evident that there is a desperate need to increase research in its cause and treatment. To prevent and eliminate the agonizing effects of Sarcoidosis, it is fundamental that the local communities, general public, health educators and medical practitioners be made more aware of its symptoms, and more knowledgeable in the process toward its relief, cure, recovery, and prevention. Sarcoidosis has been recognized by the U.S. Congress, and President Bush signed into public law a resolution proclaiming August 29, 1991, as National Sarcoidosis Awareness Day.

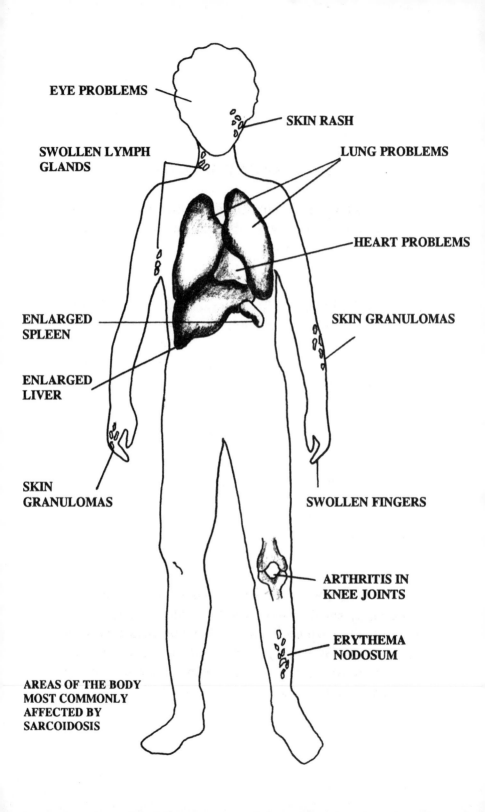

EYE PROBLEMS

SKIN RASH

SWOLLEN LYMPH
GLANDS

LUNG PROBLEMS

HEART PROBLEMS

ENLARGED
SPLEEN

SKIN GRANULOMAS

ENLARGED
LIVER

SKIN
GRANULOMAS

SWOLLEN FINGERS

ARTHRITIS IN
KNEE JOINTS

ERYTHEMA
NODOSUM

AREAS OF THE BODY
MOST COMMONLY
AFFECTED BY
SARCOIDOSIS

SIGNS AND SYMPTOMS

The following paragraphs will deal with specific "signs and symptoms", and with some of the diagnostics and treatments currently in use.

THE LUNGS - This is usually the place of "first involvement" for the Sarcoidosis patient. The belief is that it begins with alveolitis, or an inflammation of the tiny sac-like air spaces in the lungs which exchange carbon dioxide and oxygen.

THE EYES - Eye disease occurs in about 20-30% of patients, particularly frequent among children. (Although, Sarcoidosis is rarely found in children.) Any part of the eye can be affected. It can start with reddening or watery eyes. In some rare cases, cataracts, glaucoma and blindness can be a result.

THE SKIN - Twenty percent of patients are affected by small, raised patches on the face. These are occasionally purplish in color. They may also appear on the legs and be accompanied by arthritis in the ankles, elbows, wrists and hands. Erythema nodosum usually disappears, but other skin problems can persist.

THE NERVOUS SYSTEM - Occasionally, (less than 5% of the time), Sarcoidosis can lead to neurological problems. Often, patients diagnosed with Sarcoidosis who are under fifty, showed MRI findings consistent with Multiple Sclerosis and had symptoms identical to those seen in MS. Among the shared symptoms of Multiple Sclerosis and Sarcoidosis are optic-nerve abnormalities, visual disturbances, gait ataxia, incoordination, fatigue and muscle weakness.

DIAGNOSTIC TOOLS

There is no single test that can provide a diagnosis of Sarcoidosis. The first thing a doctor will do, will be to order blood work and X-rays. Dependent upon the involvement of the disease, pulmonary function tests and other tools will also be used. These tests will also enable the doctor to track the course of the disease to determine whether the patient is getting better or worse.

CHEST X-RAY

This test enables the doctor to determine the state of the lymph nodes and glands within the chest area. It can also show which area of the lungs is affected.

PULMONARY FUNCTION TESTS

This variety of tests allows the doctor to determine how well the lungs are doing their job. The lungs of Sarcoidosis patients are affected by granulomas and fibrosis of tissue which decrease the lungs capacity.

BLOOD TESTS

These are a key component to any examination. They enable the doctor to evaluate the number and types of cells in the body. They also allow him/her to measure levels of blood proteins and to reveal increases in serum calcium levels and abnormal liver function. All of these tests help to put the jigsaw puzzle of diagnosis together.

BRONCHOALVEOLAR LAVAGE

Using a bronchoscope, a long narrow tube with a light at the end, the doctor will wash out, or "lavage", cells and other materials from inside the lungs. This material is then microscopically examined and helps in diagnosis. A high number of white cells would indicate an inflammation is present.

GALLIUM SCANNING

This procedure requires the injection of a radioactive chemical element, Gallium 67. The Gallium collects in areas of the body affected by inflammation. Two days after the injection, the body is scanned for radioactivity. Since any type of inflammation will cause the Gallium to collect, a positive scan does not necessarily signal Sarcoidosis.

SLIT-LAMP EXAM

This is done with an instrument which allows a doctor to examine the inside of the eye to detect any possible damage.

Magnetic Resonance Imaging

(MRI)

Magnetic Resonance Imaging (MRI) is a new medical technology that uses the principles of magnetism; the strong magnetic field and radiowaves allow physicians to visualize certain anatomical structures more clearly than with other modalities.

The MRI was developed in the early 1980s, and was first used to image the brain and spinal cord. It has now been proved useful in diagnosing many conditions, including disorders of the brain and nervous system; bone, joint and muscle disorders; heart and blood vessel problems; and cancer of the reproductive organs, liver, kidney, lymph nodes, bladder, pancreas, and vocal cords.

The MRI produces three-dimensional appearing images of various organs and structures within the body. It also offers images that indicate how certain organs and tissues are functioning.

MRI Examination:

The primary discomfort, seems to be the claustrophobic feeling many patients suffer while lying inside the narrow, closed-in tunnel. And some patients find it extremely uncomfortable having to lie still up to fifteen minutes at a time.

In order to provide you with the best of care, you may be asked the following questions.

Do you weigh 300 pounds or more?
Can you lie flat comfortably?
Do you suffer from claustrophobia?
Are you pregnant?

Do you have any medical devices such as:

Copper-7 (IUD)?
Cardiac pacemaker?
Cerebral aneurysm clip?
Metal implants or other surgical clips?
Neurostimulators?
Hearing aid?
Do you have any metal shrapnel in your body or metal fragments in your eyes?

Advantages:

MRI do not use X-rays or any form of ionizing radiation that can be harmful to the body.

Risk factors:

Anyone with an implanted metal device such as a heart pacemaker or some surgical clips - especially those used to close blood vessels should not enter or come near a magnetic resonance imaging device. The magnetic force could cause a clip to come loose and result in hemorrhage.

Warnings have also been issued that women in their early stage of pregnancy should not be exposed to the magnetic field; there have been reports that these women have suffered headaches, swelling of the hands, and peeling of the skin.

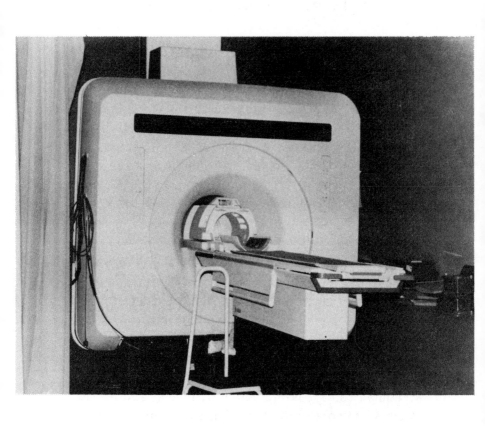

M.R.I. Machine

Sarcoidosis and The Patient

Andrew R. Freedman, M.D., F.C.C.P

Sarcoid is a very frustrating illness for physicians as well as patients. The patient often presents with the insidious onset of a constellation of symptoms that are ill-defined and seemingly disconnected. The patient can present, for example, with joint pain, chest discomfort and sweats and ultimately be subjected eventually to a series of biopsy procedures as well as testing procedures with some element of discomfort and potential complications. At the very beginning, therefore, the patient is beset by some degree of confusion and uncertainty. The physician further exacerbates the situation by attempting to convince the patient to proceed with the evaluations for the possible diagnosis and then is totally unable to furnish the patient with a satisfactory explanation for the nature of the illness. At best, the physician can say that the illness has no known etiology, an uncertain clinical presentation, a variable course, no definitive treatment, and possible measures to control the condition with complications or side effects that can actually be worse than the disease itself. Needless to say, skepticism and mistrust plague the doctor/patient relationship during the initial interaction. Furthermore, mention must be made of other illnesses which need to be considered such as tuberculosis, lymphoma, cancer, rheumatoid arthritis, lupus and even AIDS.

Patients and some physicians may vent their anger at this situation by claiming there is insufficient research, which is partially true. Attempts are being made to determine the etiology of the illness. If indeed the etiology cannot be found, certain other research tracts focus on ways to assess the activity. Nevertheless, given the incidents and prevalence of this illness, it apparently lacks the social and political flair of heart disease or elevated cholesterol levels which dominate the medical literature as well as the lay press.

Failing the ability of the medical community to solve the mysteries of sarcoid within the next two weeks, we can only content ourselves with the assiduous accumulation of descriptive data so that the manifestations of sarcoid aren't strange to us. This will certainly at least, perhaps, reduce some of the fear of sarcoid. The purpose of this sarcoid project as I perceive it from the viewpoint of physician, is to properly designate useful information to patients, physicians and those in a position of public responsibility so that all can come to grips with this, unfortunately, all too common illness. It is my sincere hope that we all keep in mind that our mutual goal is patient care and education and not the satisfaction of individual economic, social or political agendas.

Sarcoidosis and The Eye

Steven J. Faigenbaum, M.D., F.A.C.S.
Ophthalmology and Ophthalmic Surgery

Sarcoidosis is a systemic disease with unknown cause or pathogenesis. To an eye doctor it must be considered as a possible cause with just about any type of inflammatory eye condition as sarcoidosis can affect almost any part of the eye, visual system or even tissues of the orbit itself. Sarcoidosis produces a chorioretinitis type of inflammatory reaction that is hallmarked by the microscopic findings of "non-caseating epithelial cell tubercles". These epithelial cells are probably derived from the blood monocytes or the tissue histiocytes.

Most studies state that sarcoidosis involves the eye in about 20% of all cases, the lacrimal gland in 7% and the central nervous system in 4%. Lacrimal gland enlargement or dacryoadenitis may be an early finding but it is the initial manifestation in only 1% of patients.

Uveitis is the most common form of intraocular involvement in sarcoidosis. The pigmented tissue inside the eye, i.e. the iris, and the choroid are referred to as uveal tissue or the uvea. The iris alone, the choroid alone or both together may be involved. The reaction can vary from mild to severe. Usually a slit lamp exam by the ophthalmologist is needed to see the inflammatory reaction inside the eye. The symptoms of a uveitis (iritis) are generally an achy pain, light sensitivity and some blurring of vision. The symptoms however may be quite subtle and routine eye exams are needed to rule out their presence. The choroid and retina should also be examined by the ophthalmologist after the pupils have been widely dilated with drops. This should be done to all patients with known or suspected sarcoidosis. The type of inflammatory findings involving the retina are quite characteristic and look like "candle wax drippings" on the surface of this tissue.

The mucous membrane of the eye, the conjunctiva, can show small sarcoid nodule formation that can be seen also at the slit lamp in the ophthalmologist's office. A painless biopsy with topical anesthesia only can offer a tissue diagnosis in 20% or more of patients with sarcoidosis.

Some forms of sarcoidosis can also affect the brain tissue and its lining membranes as well. The optic nerve itself and the nerve that moves the muscles of the eye lid and face can be involved in this process as well. A CAT scan may be required to diagnose this involvement.

In short, sarcoidosis is a disease process that is really not that rare. The ophthalmologist can often be the first physician consulted for the presenting of symptoms.

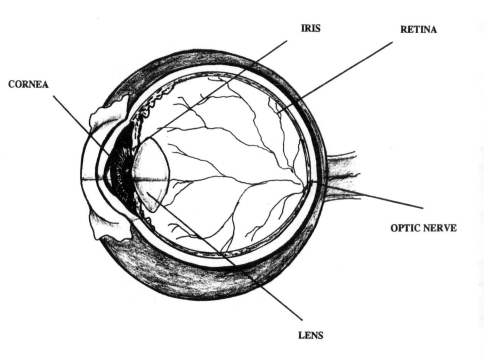

All persons with known sarcoidosis should have yearly routine eye exams even if symptom free. The ocular manifestations may vary from obvious with pain and light sensitivity to none at all. The inflammatory eye findings are usually controllable with timely diagnosis and therapy.

Sarcoid Arthritis

Nanette Alexander-Thomas, M.D.
Chief, Rheumatology Division
Harlem Hospital Center
New York City, New York

Sarcoidosis is a multisystem disease of unknown etiology that usually begins in the third or fourth decade of life. Both sexes are involved equally, but in the United States there is a higher prevalence noted in African Americans. Almost any organ can be involved, however sarcoidosis is most commonly associated with lung disease, enlarged lymph nodes, skin and eye lesions. It is characterized by noncaseating granulomas found on biopsy specimens of involved organs.

The joint disease of sarcoidosis was first described by Burman and Mayer in 1936 (1). In the majority of cases the arthritis presents with swelling, warmth and tenderness affecting several joints at the same time. They may have associated fever, however redness of the joint is not common. The most common joints affected are the ankles and knees, followed by the wrists and small joints of the hand (proximal interphalangeal joints). Inflammation of the tendons has also been noted in extreme cases can cause a Jaccoud's type arthropathy (2). This arthropathy, which is more commonly described in rheumatic fever, is characterized by severe deformities of the hands caused by inflammation of the tendons with no radiographic evidence of disease. The arthritis of sarcoidosis can occur early in the disease when it can be associated with a skin lesion called erythema nodosum, which is an inflammatory reaction. If the arthritis occurs late in the disease, the attacks are longer lasting and generally not associated with erythema nodosum. Spilbert et al (3) found that African Americans developed erythema nodosum much less frequently than Caucasians. Morning stiffness is often a prominent and long lasting symptom in patients with joint involvement. Migratory arthritis had been the usual description of early sarcoid joint disease, but in a retrospective study by Gumpel (4), this presentation was noted in only one of one hundred and eighteen patients.

Bone involvement in patients with sarcoidosis has been described (5, 6). The patient would have a similar presentation with swelling, pain and tenderness of the involved area. However, the X-ray would show "punched out" lesions, fractures and fragmentation of the bone. The frequency of osseous involvement in sarcoidosis ranges from 1 to 13%, and any bone can be involved. Of note is that the joint spaces are relatively spared and the bone lesions are asymptomatic. There is also growing evidence that sarcoid can cause a spondarthropathy (7) which is inflammation of the sacroiliac joints and associated low back pain.

Because of its relatively nonspecific presentation, sarcoid arthritis usually must be distinguished from several other diseases, most notably rheumatoid arthritis and rheumatic fever. The majority of the medical literature reviewing this topic has been done in the pediatric studies. The triad of arthritis, uveitis and rash is common to both sarcoid and rheumatoid arthritis in children. Preschool sarcoidosis is usually without pulmonary involvement thereby alleviating an important distinguishing characteristic. Discriminating features include the rash in sarcoid that is erythematous and scaly (8, 10). It does not have the evanescent pattern seen in children with juvenile rheumatoid arthritis (JRA). The intraocular changes can be distinguished by the characteristic location of inflammation in the posterior globe in sarcoid cases. The joint disease in sarcoid, in spite of dramatic swelling, will have well preserved range of motion and function, in contrast to JRA (9). Serum angiotensin converting enzyme levels were found, in a retrospective analysis of nineteen patients with sarcoid arthritis, to be elevated in 75% of patients with active sarcoid (16). The level correlated with severity of disease. It was normal in patients with rheumatoid arthritis. Finally, the radiographic appearance of patients JRA shows extensive cartilage loss and bony erosion, where X-ray changes are minimal in sarcoid. Mallory et al (11) presented four cases of children who had polyarthritis, rash and were eventually diagnosed with sarcoid after skin biopsy revealed noncaseating granulomas. They make the point that since both are diagnoses of exclusion, it is important to do tissue biopsy.

Sarcoidosis has been described as a familial disease. Blau (12, 14) presents a family of eleven members over four generations who had granulomatous disease of the skin, eyes, and joints. The disease was transmitted in an autosomal dominant fashion. Although the granulomatous findings suggest sarcoid, none of the affected family had pulmonary disease. This is thought to represent a new syndrome distinct from sarcoid because it follows simple Mendelian Inheritance. Granulomatous arthritis has been reported in a family associated with juvenile onset polyarthritis (13). It is inherited in a dominant fashion with variable penetrance. The patients also had severe hypertension and noncaseating granulomas of affected organs. Again this is a distinct entity from sarcoidosis, but along with Blau's syndrome may be part of the granulomatous disease spectrum.

These familial studies have shed some light on the etiology and inheritance of granulomatous disease. Recent immunologic research has allowed specific human genes to be identified with various diseases. Sarcoid arthritis has been linked with a class two antigen, HLA-DR3. In one study, forty two patients were identified with acute sarcoid arthritis and tissue typing was performed (14). The only antigen positively associated with sarcoid arthritis in 60% of the patients was DR3. This was corroborated by a study done by Kremer (15) who reviewed tissue typing in siblings with acute sarcoid arthritis. Future studies in these areas may help to identify the specific gene that predisposes toward disease.

Sarcoidosis is a complicated, generalized disease that may be confused with several other chronic disorders. The diagnosis can be suggested by the history and clinical presentation. Several tests can be used in addition to clarify the dilemma. Serum angiotensin converting enzyme levels should be elevated, chest X-ray in adults will show perihilar lymphadenopathy. A gallium scan, which detects areas of inflammation, will show evidence of disease in the lung, appropriate joints and possibly the parotid gland. The Kveim test is a skin test similar to that done for tuberculosis, and will be positive. Definitive diagnosis is made only after a tissue biopsy is performed and noncaseating granulomas found.

The choice of therapy depends on the severity of the disease. If the arthritis is mild, no therapy is indicated. In patients with moderately severe disease, salicylates or nonsteroidal anti-inflammatory drugs can be used. Oral colchicine has been used with success in both acute and chronic disease (17). For severe arthritis, steroids used orally, have been effective. When the inflammation has resolved, physical therapy can improve range of motion and strength in the affected joint.

References

1. **Burman, M., Mayer, L.**
   Arthroscopic examination of knee joint:
   Report of cases observed in course of
   arthroscopic examination, including
   instances of sarcoid and multiple
   polypoid fibromatosis. Arch Surg 32:846, 1936.

2. **Sukenik, S., Hendler, N. et al.**
   Jaccoud's-type arthropathy:
   An association with sarcoidosis.
   J Rheumatol 18:915-7, 1991.

3. **Spilberg, I., Siltzbach, L., McEwen, C.**
   The arthritis of sarcoidosis.
   Arth Rheum 12:126-137, 1969.

4. **Gumpel, J., Johns, C., Shulman, L.**
   The joint disease of sarcoidosis.
   Ann Rheum Dis 26:194-205, 1976

5. **Stull, M., Glass-Royal, M.**
   Musculoskeletal case of the day.
   AJR 154:1331-1336, 1990.

6. **Lemley, D., Katz, P.**
   Granulomatous musculoskeletal disease:
   sarcoidosis versus tuberculosis.
   J Rheumatol 14:1199-1201, 1987.

7. **Kirkham, B., Jobanputra, P.**
Sarcoidosis and spondarthritis.
Br J Rheumatol 27: 241-8, 1988.

8. **Lindsley, C., Godfrey, W.**
Childhood sarcoidosis manifesting
as juvenile rheumatoid arthritis.
Pediatrics 76:765-8, 1985

9. **Sahn, E., Hampton, M. et al.**
Preschool sarcoidosis masquerading as
juvenile rheumatoid arthritis: two case
reports and a review of the literature.
Ped Dermatol 7:208-213, 1990.

10. **Cassidy, J.**
Miscellaneous conditions associated
with arthritis in children.
Ped Clin North Am 33:1033-1052, 1986.

11. **Mallory, S., Paller, A. Et al.**
Sarcoidosis in children: differentiation
from juvenile rheumatoid arthritis.
Ped Dermatol 4: 313-319, 1987.

12. **Blau, E.**
Familial granulomatous arthritis, iritis,
and rash. J. Pediatr 107:689-693, 1985.

13. Rotenstein, D., Gibbas, D. Et Al.
    Familial granulomatous arthritis with
    polyarthritis of juvenile onset.
    N Engl J Med 306:86-90, 1982

14. Krause, A., Goebel, K.
    Class 2 MHC antigen (HLA-DR3)
    predisposes to sarcoid arthritis.
    J Clin Lab Immunol 24:25-27, 1987.

15. Kremer, J.
    Histologic findings in siblings with
    acute sarcoid arthritis: association
    with the B8, DR3 phenotype.
    J Rheumatol 13:593-7, 1986.

16. Sequeira, W., Stinar, D.
    Serum angiotensin-converting
    enzyme levels in sarcoid arthritis.
    Arch Intern Med 146:125-7, 1986.

17. Rubinstein, I., Baum, G.
    Colchicine therapy in sarcoid
    arthropathy.
    Pediatr 78:717-8, 1986.

JOINTS

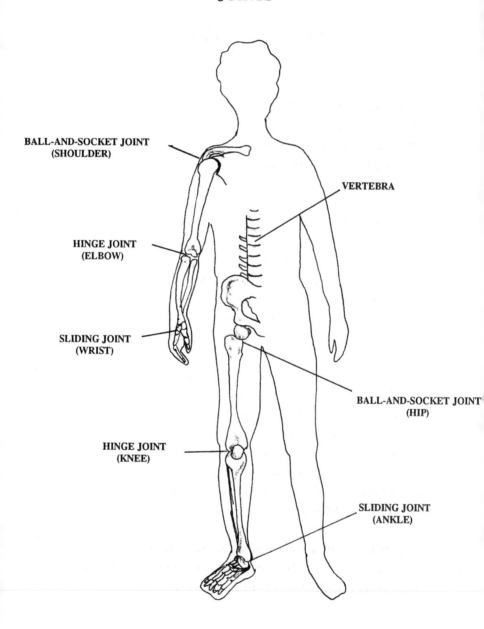

BALL-AND-SOCKET JOINT
(SHOULDER)

VERTEBRA

HINGE JOINT
(ELBOW)

SLIDING JOINT
(WRIST)

BALL-AND-SOCKET JOINT
(HIP)

HINGE JOINT
(KNEE)

SLIDING JOINT
(ANKLE)

Neurosarcoidosis

Thomas F. Scott, M.D.
Assistant Professor of the
Medical College of Pennsylvania
at Allegheny General Hospital

Although one usually thinks of lungs when dealing with sarcoidosis, actually many other systems, including the central nervous system (that is the brain and spinal cord), peripheral nervous system (the nerves after they have left the spinal cord), muscles, and eye may all be affected by sarcoidosis, and may lead a patient to be referred to a neurologist. The nervous system is affected in about 1 out of 20 patients with sarcoidosis. The symptoms can relapse and remit, and occasionally patients have been misdiagnosed as having multiple sclerosis because of the similarity between the relapsing and remitting symptoms of these two diseases. Sarcoidosis may affect any part of the nervous system, and thus may give any imaginable type of nervous system problem, including weakness, numbness, problems with coordination, and even psychiatric problems.

The involvement of nervous tissues in this disease is somewhat complicated, and more remains to be learned. However, it is known that in many patients the reason for the patient's symptoms are related to the formation of granulomas (tumor like nodules of inflammatory tissue, which are the hallmark of sarcoidosis) within the nervous system. These granulomas may push away normal tissue, and cause pressure, and hence dysfunction. Blood flow may also be interrupted by compression or by involvement of small arteries with granulomatous inflammation.

Because this particular problem of nervous system dysfunction in patients with sarcoidosis is usually treatable, patients with these problems should seek help from physicians for diagnosis and treatment.

There has been an improvement in physicians' ability to diagnose neurosarcoidosis, thanks mostly to new technology. Probably the most important new technology is the magnetic resonance scanner (MRI - Magnetic Resonance Imaging). This is a type of computerized imaging of the body's interior, which is very sensitive for detecting sarcoid changes within the nervous system. Almost all patients with symptoms referable to brain dysfunction (such as visual problems, numbness, weakness) will have abnormalities on their MRI scan. CT scan (computerized tomography) is somewhat less sensitive but can also be useful. Improvement has also been made in detecting peripheral nerve problems.

Electrical tests can be done on the nerves in the arms and legs (electromyography) which may detect sarcoid involvement of the nerves in the arms and legs. Similar electrical testing can also detect sarcoid within muscle tissue. A third technology, involving improved study of spinal fluid, can also help detect evidence of active sarcoidosis in the central nervous system. In order to do this type of testing, a spinal tap (lumbar puncture) must be performed.

These new technologies are important, since identifying neurosarcoidosis early may lead to early treatment and hence less disability over the long run. Problems in the nervous system, as in lungs, tend to respond to steroids. If steroids fail, newer drugs or even radiotherapy has been used with success. About one third to one half of patients with neurologic sarcoidosis will have a relapsing course, so long term follow up with a neurologist may become necessary.

Symptoms

Visual

Loss of vision or blurred vision, double vision.

Motor System:

Weakness, trouble with coordination and walking, trouble with writing or manipulating fine objects.

Sensory system:

Numbness, tingling, inability to sense heat or textures, burning sensations, pain.

Other:
(possibly suggestive of neurologic damage)

Headaches, stiff neck, fatigue, lack of endurance, bladder dysfunction, incontinence.

SARCOIDOSIS AND THE HEART

Luther T. Clark, M.D.

Sarcoidosis is a multisystemic disease of unknown etiology. The heart is involved in twenty to thirty percent of patients with generalized sarcoidosis although symptoms of cardiac involvement occur in less than 5 percent of cases. The most common symptoms of cardiac involvement of patients with sarcoidosis are congestive heart failure, heart block, premature ventricular contractions (extra heart beats), rapid heart beat, and pericarditis. Rarely, patients may present with symptoms suggesting a heart attack.

The most common form of heart disease in patients with sarcoidosis is that resulting from severe pulmonary disease. When the lungs are severely affected with granulomas and fibrosis, the resulting elevation of blood pressures in the lungs may cause impairment of right ventricular function. Following cardiac involvement, symptoms may be present for variable lengths of time, but usually they are progressive and may show only a limited response to therapy.

The diagnosis of cardiac sarcoidosis is usually suspected on clinical grounds and supported by findings on the electrocardiogram, chest X-ray, and cardiac scan. Occasionally, a biopsy of the heart may be required for diagnosis.

Treatment depends on the nature of the cardiac involvement. Arrhythmias may respond to anti-arrhythmic medications. Corticosteroids may be of benefit in some patients with arrhythmias, conduction disturbances, or congestive heart failure. Patients with severe heart block may require a pacemaker.

Sarcoidosis and Its' Symptoms

Sarcoidosis is a multisystemic disease, whose symptoms often mimics many other diseases. There are no answers as to why some patients may exhibit little or no symptoms; while others may experience some of the symptoms listed below. On the following pages, are illustrations of other possible areas of involvement.

persistent coughing
low grade fever
night sweats
chest pains
difficulty breathing
shortness of breath
stiff neck
tinnitus
migraines
weight loss
kidney problems
enlarged liver
joint pain-knees, wrists, fingers
leg cramps
muscle weakness-arms, hands, legs

fatigue
rapid heart beat
dizziness
sinusitis
seizures
swollen legs/ankles
coordination
balance
abdominal pain
enlarged spleen
swollen lymph glands
nausea
psychosis
Bell's Palsy
footdrop
walking, &
walking up stairs

depression
incontinence

Vision:
blurred vision,
loss of vision,
light sensitivity,
dry eyes

Skin:
dry, flaky patches,
rash (red bumps),
skin discolorations,
tissue scarring

NERVOUS SYSTEM

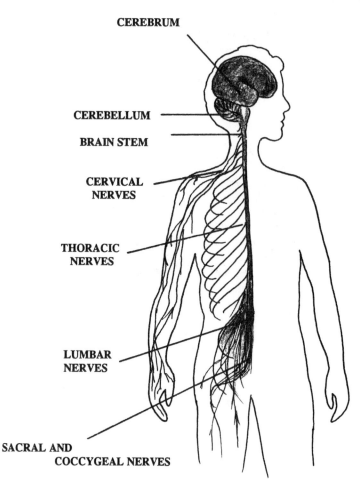

CEREBRUM

CEREBELLUM

BRAIN STEM

CERVICAL
NERVES

THORACIC
NERVES

LUMBAR
NERVES

SACRAL AND
COCCYGEAL NERVES

THE BRAIN

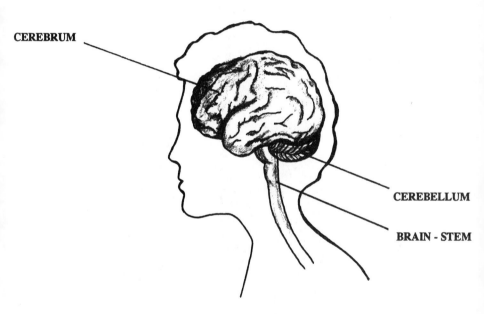

CEREBRUM

CEREBELLUM

BRAIN - STEM

RESPIRATORY

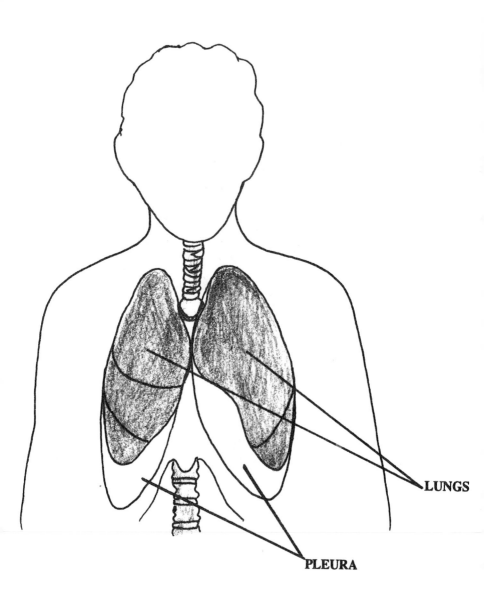

LUNGS

PLEURA

THE HEART

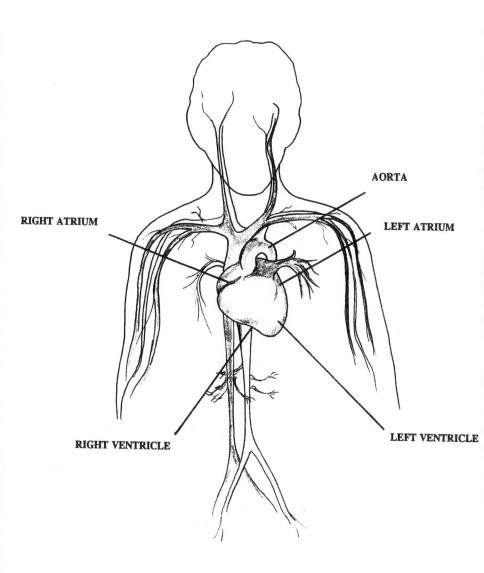

AORTA

RIGHT ATRIUM

LEFT ATRIUM

RIGHT VENTRICLE

LEFT VENTRICLE

LYMPHATIC SYSTEM

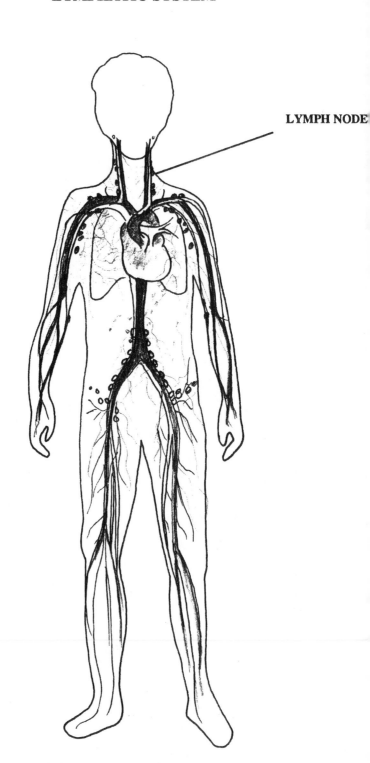

LYMPH NODE

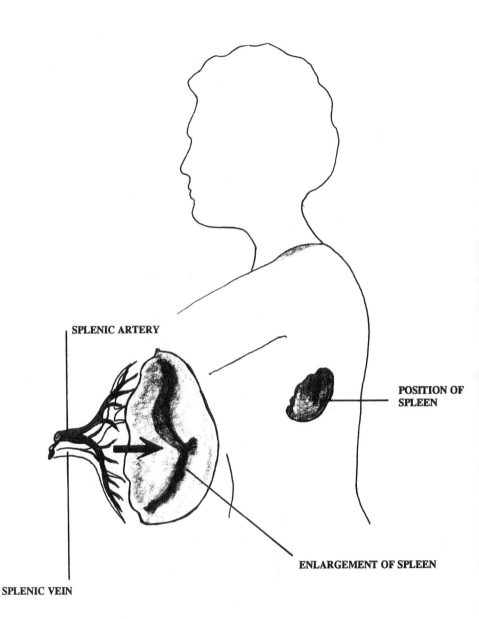

SPLENIC ARTERY

POSITION OF
SPLEEN

ENLARGEMENT OF SPLEEN

SPLENIC VEIN

SPLEEN

CIRCULATORY SYSTEM

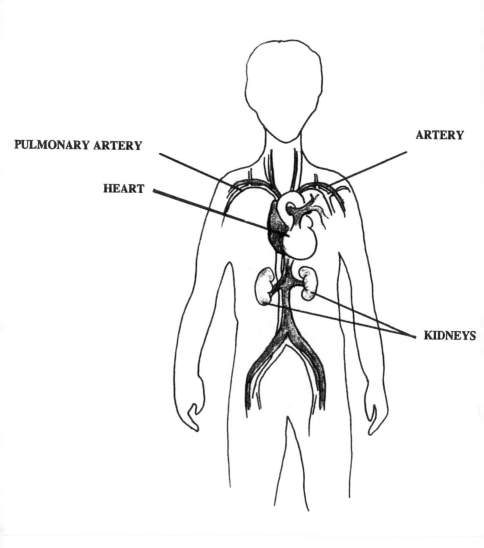

PULMONARY ARTERY

ARTERY

HEART

KIDNEYS

DIGESTIVE SYSTEM

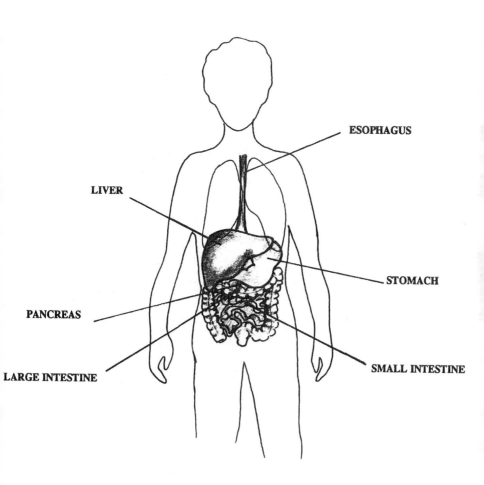

ESOPHAGUS

LIVER

STOMACH

PANCREAS

SMALL INTESTINE

LARGE INTESTINE

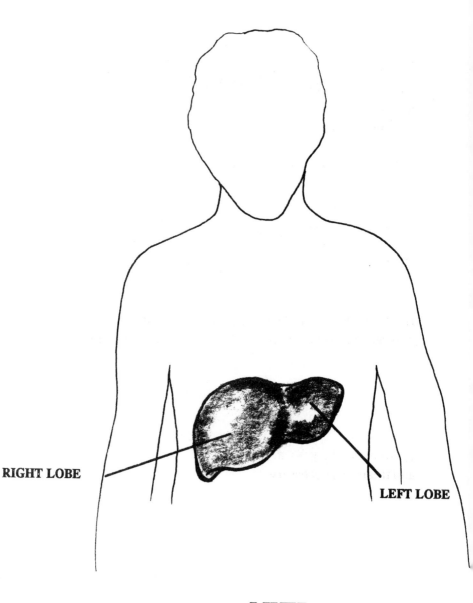

RIGHT LOBE

LEFT LOBE

LIVER

Management

No one yet knows what causes Sarcoidosis. So there are no known cures or preventive measures at this time. It is recommended that you should;

- Follow sensible health habits

- Don't smoke

- Avoid exposure to other substances such as dusts and chemicals that are harmful to your lungs

If you have Sarcoidosis, the best medical professional will be a lung specialist or a doctor with a special interest in the disease, itself.

Sarcoidosis is a life long disease, and it would be smart to have regular physical and eye checkups. If you have symptoms, see your doctor, so that you may be watched and treated as necessary.

If you are planning to have a baby, discuss the possibilities with your doctor. Sarcoidosis does not usually affect the fetus or baby in any way.

Keep in touch with others with the disease. There are organizations and support groups to help you to help yourself.

IDEAS AND CONSIDERATIONS FOR STARTING A SELF-HELP MUTUAL AID GROUP FOR SARCOIDOSIS

A self-help group can offer persons with Sarcoidosis an opportunity to meet with others and share their experiences, knowledge, strengths and hopes. Run by, and for their members, a self-help group can be described as a "mutual help" group since members are helping one another. Dozens of different self-help groups are started each week across the nation by ordinary people with a little bit of courage, a fair sense of commitment, and a heavy amount of caring. The following guidelines are based on experiences at the Self-Help Clearinghouse, helping hundreds of individuals to start different groups. While there is no one recipe for starting a group (you will be looking at local resources and members' specific needs), we have listed below a few general considerations you may find helpful.

1. Do not try to Re-invent the Wheel.

If you are interested in starting a Sarcoidosis group, talk to people who are involved in groups now or have started ones before. Check with your Sarcoidosis Resource Center to find out about existing groups. Contact some of those groups by phone or mail. Ask for any sample materials they have -- flyers, brochures, newsletters, press releases, or other printed material.

If you have a local self-help clearing house in your area, determine what help they can provide you in developing a group. Consider attending a few meetings of other types of self-help groups to get a feel for how they operate--then borrow what you consider their best techniques and formats to use in your own group.

2. Think "Mutual-Help" From the Start.

Find a few others who share your interest in starting, (not simply joining) a self-help group. Put out flyers or letters that specifically cite this. Your "core group" or "steering committee" can help prevent you from "burning out". But perhaps more importantly, if several people are involved in the planning and initial tasks (refreshments, publicity, name tags, greeters, etc.), they will be role models for others at the time of the first public meeting. They will demonstrate what self-help mutual aid is all about -- not one person doing it all, but a group effort. Try to enlist the aid of professionals who may see Sarcoidosis patients. Ask if they would refer to you any patients who may be interested in helping to start a group. Ask those same professionals if they would be willing to speak before any group that is eventually started.

3. Find a Suitable Meeting Place and Time.
Try to obtain free meeting space at a local church,
synagogue, library, community center, hospital or social
service agency. The facilities should be barrier free. If
you anticipate a small group and feel more comfortable
with the idea, consider initial meetings in members'
homes. Would evening or day meetings be better for
members? Most prefer weeknights. It is easier for people
to remember the meeting time if it's a regular day of the
week or month, like the second Thursday of the month,
etc. Some people like to have the meeting around an
informal supper, such as a potluck. A few even have
meetings at a diner or restaurant.

4. Publicizing and Running your first Meeting.

Reaching potential members is never easy. Consider
where people with Sarcoidosis would go. Wouldn't they
be seen by particular doctors or at pulmonary clinics at
local hospitals? Contacting physicians and other health
professionals (e.g., local Lung Associations) can be one
approach to try. Flyers in post offices, hospitals, and
libraries may help. Free announcements in the
community calendar sections of local newspapers can be
especially fruitful. Better yet, try phoning the editor, and
simply explain what type of group you want to start.
Indicate how you would like to reach out to other people

who have this condition, while educating the public to the problem. Be prepared with some facts on the disorder that can be expressed in nonmedical terms. Also consider providing the names of physicians or health professionals who know about Sarcoidosis and would be willing to speak to a reporter. Remember to clear the use of their names with them before using them as spokespersons.

The first meeting should be arranged so that there will be ample time for you to describe your interests and your work, while allowing others the opportunity to share their feelings and concerns. Do those attending agree that such a group is needed? Will they attend another meeting, helping out as needed? What would they like to see the group do, what issues discussed or presented? Based on members' needs, interests, and responses, make plans for your next meeting.

5. Future Meetings.

Other considerations for future meetings may be the following:

a. Defining the purpose of the group - to provide education and support? This may be added to any flyer or brochure you have for the group. Include guidelines or agenda you have for your meetings.

b. Membership. Who can attend meetings? Should regular membership be limited to those with Sarcoidosis with an associate membership for spouses, other family members and friends?

c. Meeting format. What combination of discussion time, education, business meeting, service planning, socializing, etc. suits your group best? What guidelines might you use to assure that discussion be nonjudgemental, confidential and informative? Topics can be selected or guest speakers invited. A good discussion group size is seven to fifteen. As your meeting grows larger, consider breaking down into smaller groups for discussion.

d. Phone network. Self-help groups should provide an atmosphere of caring, sharing and support when needed. Many groups encourage the exchange of telephone numbers to provide help over the phone whenever it is needed.

e. Use of professionals. Consider using professionals as speakers, advisors, consultants to your groups, and sources of continued referrals.

f. Projects. Always begin with small projects. Rejoice and pat yourselves on the back when you succeed with these first projects, like having a flyer or a brochure printed, or developing a library or service project. Then, with time, work your way up to the more difficult tasks.

g. Lastly, expect your group to experience "Up's and Down's" in terms of attendance and enthusiasm. Such fluctuations are natural and to be expected. You may want to consider joining or forming a coalition or a group of leaders, for periodic mutual support and the sharing of program ideas and successes.

For more ideas & detailed information on starting a group, consider getting one of the following:

Hill, Karen (with update by Hector Balthazar). Helping You Helps Me: A Guide Book for Self-Help Groups. 1986, 82 pages. Order for $4.50 from Canadian Council on Social Development, Attn: Publications, P.O. Box 3505, Station C, Ottawa, Ontario; Canada K1Y 4G1.

Humm, Andy How to organize a Self-Help Group. 1979, 48 pages. Order for $6.00 each from the National Self-Help Clearinghouse, 25 West 43rd Street, New York, New York 10036

SOCIAL SECURITY DISABILITY AND YOU

Probably the single factor most influential to the success of your application or appeal is the quality of medical documentation and support obtained from your primary physician.

It is crucial that your primary physician be an effective clinician, familiar with Sarcoidosis and its many idiosyncrasies. In addition, the physician must believe you are medically disabled and be willing to advance your claim strongly to the SSA. The importance of strong, convincing medical support from the treating physician(s) cannot be overestimated. It will be almost impossible to obtain eligibility without it.

The doctor will be asked to file reports and send records to the SSA for review. He or she may also need to sign affidavits and/or appear as a witness at later hearings in order for you to obtain or maintain eligibility. (Other doctors who have treated you, as well as hospitals that have admitted you for treatment, will also be asked to submit forms and reports.)

Some physicians may be more willing than others to discuss and be supportive of your non-clinical interests, such as insurance and benefits. Check with your primary physician in advance of filing a claim. If it seems that he or she is not prepared to give you the kind of support you think you will need, consider your options carefully.

Make sure your doctor is familiar with Social Security "medical listing" in general, and the specific listing for Sarcoidosis. Is the doctor aware of the combined effect of multiple impairments? Does the physician understand how best to structure a report for Social Security purposes?

If your doctor is unfamiliar with Sarcoidosis, or if he or she is unfamiliar with Social Security policies, procedures, and forms, this can create a serious problem for you. It is important to meet with the physician before his or her report is prepared, to review Social Security disability standards and those aspects of your illness and its consequences that need to be stressed.

Some actions can be taken to correct or clarify an application or appeal that has already been submitted. These include: developing new medical evidence; challenging consultative opinions; bringing in lay or expert witnesses to establish your demonstrated capacity in work settings, your vocational abilities, and your future employability.

Medical Documentation

Keep your physician fully informed about your condition, including any new symptoms or exacerbations, and their effects on your life at home and at work. Request that these be made part of your medical record. The content of your medical record, like the quality of your physician's support, will be crucial to your success.

Keep an accurate diary of all symptoms, experiences, facts, events, and conversations at work and elsewhere, that strike you as important indicators of your illness and its effects. The diary entries may help you to remember things you wish to tell your physician for the record. The diary may itself be introduced as documentary support of any claim that you may make.

If you are found to meet the preliminary eligibility requirements for either SSDI or SSI, your file will be sent to your state agency responsible for determining medical disability. This agency is usually referred to as the Disability Determination Service (DDS). The agency develops each individual claimant's medical evidence by obtaining information from doctors and hospitals listed in the Social Security benefit application.

If the hospitals and doctors do not respond, the DDS may make its decision without this evidence. Thus, it is very important for you to make sure that these sources respond to these requests for information where you expect their responses to be supportive. Also, ensure that their reports are submitted in a timely fashion.

If, after examining the available medical evidence, the DDS feels it needs more information to make a decision, it may schedule you to receive an additional medical examination or review known as a "consultative examination". (Please note: a person with a disability is entitled to travel reimbursement for attending a consultative examination. This can be obtained in advance if you need it.) Refusal to participate in this examination without good cause may result in a denial of eligibility.

The type of examination and/or test(s) purchased for the consultative examination will depend upon the specific information the DDS evaluator feels is necessary.

The consultative examiner's findings are sent to DDS doctors who review the information along with the rest of the file and make a decision on the disability claim in conjunction with the rest of the disability evaluation team.

DDS then notifies the SSA Office of Disability Operations (The ODO, located in Baltimore, Maryland) of its decision. The ODO notifies the claimant of the results of the process.

You need to be aware that the findings of a consultative examination are not necessarily final. There have been successful appeals of benefit denials based partly on inadequacies in the consultative examinations performed. (For example, there are cases in which SSA consultant physicians have been found not to have performed examinations of claimants, but rather have simply based their results on reviews of records.)

Wherever appropriate, (such as in an appeal hearing), introduce authoritative documentation concerning Sarcoidosis. Many useful items are available from the National offices of the Sarcoidosis Foundation and the Sarcoidosis Resource Center.

INFORMATION TO BRING WHEN
APPLYING FOR SSDI AND SSI

You can speed up your claim if you have this information when you contact the Social Security Office:

SOCIAL SECURITY NUMBERS

* Yours, your spouse's and any other dependent:
* Any other number on which you or dependents receive or received Social Security checks.

ABOUT YOUR ILLNESS

* What it is and when it started;
* How it keeps you from working;
* Date you stopped working;
* If you returned to work, give date, employer, and information about your current job.

MEDICAL INFORMATION

* List complete names, addresses, and phone numbers of all doctors, hospitals, or other medical facilities where you were treated or tested.

* Dates of medical visits and type of treatment or tests;

* Hospital, clinic and/or Medicaid number;

* Claim number for any other disability checks you receive or have applied for.

* Medicines you now take: Names, dosage, how often;

* Any restrictions your doctor placed on you.

BRING ANY MEDICAL REPORTS OR
PRESCRIPTIONS YOU HAVE.

They will be copied and returned.

YOUR RESPONSIBILITY

It is your responsibility, and in your best interest, to cooperate fully in providing any information requested.

Do not delay filing a claim if you do not yet have the information shown here. The people at the Social Security Office will help you.

IN ADDITION

If you are applying for SSI you should also bring the following:

* The latest tax bill or assessment notice if you own real estate other than your home.

* Bank book, insurance policies, burial plot or burial fund records,and other papers that show your resources.

Appeals

In the event your claim is denied, you may file an appeal. If you attend an appeal hearing or have some other personal meeting at the Social Security office, do not try to look especially healthy or attractive. Look the way you feel.

In many cases, an Administrative Law Judge's decision is influenced by the claimant's appearance. Experience suggests that many people who have a disabling illness nevertheless make a good appearance. Part of the reason is that some of the symptoms of Sarcoidosis, such as pain or fatigue, are "invisible." In addition, some people try to overcompensate to make a good appearance, even though they feel poorly.

Similarly, do not act the part of a hero by playing down your limitations or exaggerating your capacities. If you indicate on forms or in other ways that you can do sedentary work, your application or appeal will very likely be denied.

Although you should definitely be polite and reasonably cooperative, it is wrong to think that overstating your functional capacity and "braving it out" will favorably impress the Social Security staff or consultative physicians and cause them to make a sympathetic report or reach a more favorable decision in your case than they otherwise would. You may simply be undercutting your own chances of obtaining benefits that you may need and for which you should be eligible.

The Appeal Process

1. Reconsideration:
   Apply within 60 days after denial.

Applicants can ask to have their application reconsidered. New medical evidence to update the applicants file must be submitted. The updated file will be given to an examiner and doctor.

2. Hearing before an Administrative Law Judge:
   Apply within 60 days after reconsideration denial.

The Administrative Law Judge reviews updated records and conducts a hearing. Applicants have the right to produce witnesses, and be represented by a lawyer, or other qualified representative.

3. Appeals Court Review:
   Apply within 60 days after the hearing.

The decision of the Administrative Law Judge can be reviewed by a 15 member Social Security Appeals Council. Request for review must be made within 60 days after denial by the Administrative Law Judge.

If the council agrees to review the claim, it may agree or disagree with the Administrative Law Judge's action, or it may send the case back to the Administrative Law Judge for reconsideration.

4. Federal Court Appeal:
When Social Security closes case.

If the Appeals Council denies the disability claim or refuses to review it, the case can then be taken to the Federal Courts.

Rights

1. Representation by a lawyer or other appropriate advocate.

2. Access to records and addition of relevant information.

3. Applicants may select their own witnesses.

Attorneys and Other Advocates

In preparation for a hearing on appeal of an SSA decision, you (the attorney or advocate) may wish to:

--Interview the claimant.

--Contact the Sarcoidosis Foundation to obtain general information about Sarcoidosis.

--Review the claimant's file at the office of Hearings and Appeals, and obtain copies of relevant documents.

--Obtain all available medical evidence, including hospital and clinic records, and reports and letters from treating doctors, psychiatrists, counselors and others. Obtain all available vocational evidence, including employment records, and testimony by former employers, employees, and co-workers.

--Seek out friends, family, members, neighbors and others who might be willing to offer evidence by affidavit or as live witnesses concerning the effects of this disability on the claimant's life, including their observations of its limiting effects on his or her ability to work. While this kind of evidence will not be the sole basis for establishing disability, it can favorably impress a judge with the claimant's diligence and good faith.

--Be prepared to show that the claimant has cooperated with any vocational rehabilitation workers who have been involved with the claimant. The SSA can refer claimants for an evaluation of vocational potentials and for job retraining by the state's Department of Vocational Rehabilitation. Failure of a claimant to participate in the evaluation/retraining process can result in termination of benefits by the SSA. (It should be noted though that a referral to the state agency is not always made.)

--Prepare yourself, the claimant, and witnesses for the testimony that will be given at the hearing. For example, be clear about the specific disabilities and limitations you intend to establish and what specific examples from the claimant's daily life and work activities are to be discussed to demonstrate these limitations.

--Prepare the claimant for ALJ hearing by reviewing beforehand the typical questions asked by an ALJ.

--These may include:

Describing a normal day from getting up in the morning until going to bed at night.

Describing performance of routine tasks such as grocery shopping.

Indicating whether claimant drives an automobile and, if so, for how long and under what circumstances.

Features of the disease that you may wish to emphasize include fatigue, the fact that in many instances, the disease is characterized by exacerbations and remissions; the progressive or incremental nature of Sarcoidosis; the possibility of incremental residual impairments following each exacerbation; the fact that it is lifelong; its incurability; the attendant difficulties of adapting and readapting to each new change and to the tremendous variety of symptoms; and the fact that there is no effective treatment to alter the course of the disease. If you introduce written materials on these subjects, make sure they are sent to the ALJ prior to hearing.

Following is a list of useful legal principles for representing a claimant with Sarcoidosis.

-- The ALJ is required to take into consideration "non-exertional impairments" in determining whether a claimant is disabled. Persons with Sarcoidosis may suffer from a variety of non-exertional impairments that should be emphasized at the hearing.

--The ALJ must consider the combined effects
   of multiple impairments.

--The shifting burden of proof.

After you prove that the claimant is unable to return to his
or her past work, the burden shifts to the SSA to
demonstrate that jobs are available that the claimant can
perform.

This places a heavy burden on the SSA, particularly if you
can prove that the claimant is unable to return to his or her
past job because of extreme fatigue. For example, show
that the claimant requires rest after 15 minutes to one-half
hour of activity. Is there any job available to a person with
such an impairment?

INADEQUATE REPRESENTATION AT THE ADMINISTRATIVE LAW JUDGE LEVEL.

More frequently than not, a disabled claimant is unrepresented before the Administrative Law Judge. Notwithstanding the case law on the matter, the Administrative Law Judges frequently fail to fully develop the record. They do not adequately examine the claimant and claimants' witnesses. The ALJs usually uncritically accept the hospital and medical reports as prepared, and ignore the ambiguities and uncertainties in the records.

The rate of reversals of an ALJ in Social Security matters continues to be higher than in any other area of the law. The decisions of the Courts of Appeal are often ignored. Whether this is because the Administrative Law Judges are overworked or over-supervised by the Secretary's office (Secretary of Health and Human Services), however, is hard to tell. It is difficult to believe that the Administrative Law Judges, as a group, lack care and compassion. It would seem, that they would apply the decisions of various Courts of Appeal if they had the time to do so and were permitted to do so.

Therefore, it is extremely important that claimants have representation at the Administrative Law Judge level so that the record can be fully and fairly developed.

THE CLARITY OF HOSPITAL AND MEDICAL RECORDS

Time after time, the Court receives administrative records which contain hospital and medical reports which cannot be read. The Administrative Law Judge and the Secretary have based decisions on illegible records. In this regard, the Courts have uniformly held that the Secretary has the responsibility of preparing records that it intends to rely on, and the claimants and their lawyers have a right to insist that the reports be prepared in a readable form. The Secretary resists, the United States Attorney resists, and the hospitals and doctors resist; but the price of an unreadable record is often a denial of benefits. As far as the court is concerned, when the records are not readable, the United States Attorney is required to furnish readable copies.

MEDICAL REPORTS

There is perhaps nothing more annoying to the court than a record with hospital and medical reports which contain either no opinions as to disability, or contradictory ones. This is particularly annoying where no effort has been made before the Administrative Law Judge to resolve the ambiguities or contradictions. Rather than have a claimant lose a good case, it is important that the hospital and medical records be clarified by interrogatories, depositions or evidentiary hearings if there is no other way to accomplish this end. Moreover, be sure that the testimony of your claimant is clear and to the point.

LOCAL SOCIAL SECURITY OFFICE

Contact Person:

_____

Address:

_____

_____

Phone: _____

LAWYER

Name:

_____

Address:

_____

_____

Phone: _____

Government

On August 14, 1991

The President of the United States

signed into public law

The House Joint Resolution 309

Proclaiming

August 29, 1991

National Sarcoidosis Awareness Day

Public Law 102-94
102d Congress

Joint Resolution

Aug. 14, 1991
[H.J. Res. 309]

Designating August 29, 1991, as "National Sarcoidosis Awareness Day".

Whereas sarcoidosis is a systemic disease of unknown causes that can affect any part of the body;

Whereas sarcoidosis affects between 20 and 50 individuals in 100,000 in the United States;

Whereas most victims of the disease range in age between 20 and 40 years, with blacks being affected at least 10 times more often than other ethnic groups in the United States;

Whereas between 10 to 20 percent of individuals stricken with sarcoidosis eventually develop serious disabling conditions caused by damage to vital organs, such as lungs, heart, and central nervous system;

Whereas sarcoidosis is an enigma in the realm of medicine and disease that requires extensive and ongoing study and research in an effort to develop an effective treatment and eventually a cure;

Whereas individuals with sarcoidosis and family members across the United States are seeking treatment and support services to assist in controlling the effects of the disease;

Whereas grassroot support groups and nonprofit organizations are forming across the United States to encourage public awareness of the mysterious and debilitating disease;

Whereas the Federal Government has a responsibility to lead a nationwide effort to find a cure for the disabling disease; and

Whereas the Federal Government should make research into the causes of the life-threatening ailment a greater priority and provide the public with more information about potential treatments for individuals with sarcoidosis: Now, therefore, be it

Resolved by the Senate and House of Representatives of the United States of America in Congress assembled, That August 29, 1991, is designated as "National Sarcoidosis Awareness Day", and the President is authorized and requested to issue a proclamation calling upon the people of the United States to observe the week with appropriate ceremonies and activities.

Approved August 14, 1991.

LEGISLATIVE HISTORY—H.J. Res. 309:

CONGRESSIONAL RECORD, Vol. 137 (1991):
    Aug. 1, considered and passed House.
    Aug. 2, considered and passed Senate.

O

National Sarcoidosis Awareness Day, 1991

By the President of the United States of America

A Proclamation

Sarcoidosis, a disease that affects many of our fellow citizens and people around the world, remains shrouded in mystery. Skin-related symptoms of this chronic, multi-system disease were first recognized more than 100 years ago; however, the effects of sarcoidosis on other bodily organs were not observed until the first quarter of this century. Today researchers are still trying to learn more about the cause and the nature of this affliction.

Sarcoidosis can strike people of all races and of all ages, but, according to the United States Department of Health and Human Services, it is most common among black Americans who are between the ages of 20 and 40. While no cause has yet been identified, it is thought that heredity predisposes some individuals to the disease. Intensive research during the past decade has not only supported this belief but also enabled physicians to diagnose and to manage sarcoidosis more effectively.

Today researchers at both the National Institute of Allergy and Infectious Diseases and the National Heart, Lung, and Blood Institute are leading studies on the etiology, diagnosis, and treatment of sarcoidosis. On this occasion, we recognize their work and that of other concerned physicians and scientists throughout the United States. We also salute the victims of sarcoidosis who demonstrate great courage and determination in their efforts to cope with the disease; and we pay tribute to their family members and to other concerned Americans who are engaged in grass-roots efforts to promote awareness of sarcoidosis, as well as improved treatment and support for its victims.

To focus national attention on sarcoidosis, the Congress, by House Joint Resolution 309, has designated August 29, 1991, as "National Sarcoidosis Awareness Day" and has authorized and requested the President to issue a proclamation in observance of this day.

NOW, THEREFORE, I, GEORGE BUSH, President of the United States of America, do hereby proclaim August 29, 1991, as National Sarcoidosis Awareness Day. I invite all Americans to join in observing this day with appropriate programs and activities.

IN WITNESS WHEREOF, I have hereunto set my hand this fifteenth day of August, in the year of our Lord nineteen hundred and ninety-one, and of the Independence of the United States of America the two hundred and sixteenth.

Ay Bush

102D CONGRESS
1ST SESSION

H. J. RES. 309

Designating August 29, 1991, as "National Sarcoidosis Awareness Day".

IN THE HOUSE OF REPRESENTATIVES

JULY 18, 1991

Mr. SLATTERY (for himself, Mr. ACKERMAN, Mr. ALEXANDER, Mr. ASPIN, Mr. BARNARD, Mr. BATEMAN, Mr. BENNETT, Mr. BEVILL, Mr. BILBRAY, Mr. BILIRAKIS, Mr. BLILEY, Mr. BONIOR, Mr. BORSKI, Mrs. BOXER, Mr. BROOKS, Mr. BUSTAMANTE, Mr. CALLAHAN, Mr. CARR, Mr. CARPER, Mr. CHAPMAN, Mr. CLEMENT, Mr. CONYERS, Mr. COOPER, Mr. COUGHLIN, Mr. DAVIS, Mr. DELLUMS, Mr. DWYER of New Jersey, Mr. ECKART, Mr. EMERSON, Mr. ERDREICH, Mr. ESPY, Mr. FALEOMAVAEGA, Mr. FAZIO, Mr. FISH, Mr. FORD of Michigan, Mr. FROST, Mr. GEREN of Texas, Mr. GOODLING, Mr. GORDON, Mr. GRANDY, Mr. GUARINI, Mr. HARRIS, Mr. HATCHER, Mr. HAYES of Illinois, Mr. HAYES of Louisiana, Mr. HEFNER, Mr. HOCHBRUECKNER, Mr. HORTON, Mr. HUBBARD, Mr. JACOBS, Mr. JOHNSON of South Dakota, Mr. KASICH, Mr. KOLTER, Mr. LAGOMARSINO, Mr. LANCASTER, Mr. LANTOS, Mr. LAUGHLIN, Mr. LEHMAN of Florida, Mr. LEWIS of Georgia, Mr. LIVINGSTON, Ms. LONG, Mr. McCLOSKEY, Mr. McCOLLUM, Mr. McDADE, Mr. McDERMOTT, Mr. McGRATH, Mr. McHUGH, Mr. McMILLEN of Maryland, Mr. McNULTY, Mr. MARKEY, Mr. MARTIN, Mr. MARTINEZ, Mr. MAVROULES, Mrs. MEYERS of Kansas, Mr. MFUME, Mrs. MORELLA, Mr. MURTHA, Mr. NEAL of Massachusetts, Mr. NEAL of North Carolina, Ms. OAKAR, Mr. OWENS of New York, Mr. OWENS of Utah, Mr. PALLONE, Mr. PANETTA, Mrs. PATTERSON, Mr. PAYNE of New Jersey, Ms. PELOSI, Mr. PICKETT, Mr. PRICE, Mr. PURSELL, Mr. QUILLEN, Mr. RANGEL, Mr. RAVENEL, Mr. RINALDO, Mr. ROBERTS, Mr. ROE, Mrs. ROUKEMA, Mr. ROWLAND, Mr. ROYBAL, Mr. SAVAGE, Mr. SERRANO, Mr. SMITH of Florida, Mr. SOLOMON, Mr. SPENCE, Mr. SPRATT, Mr. STAGGERS, Mr. STENHOLM, Mr. STUMP, Mr. TALLON, Mr. TAUZIN, Mr. TRAFICANT, Mrs. UNSOELD, Mr. VALENTINE, Mr. WALSH, Mr. WAXMAN, Mr. WEBER, Mr. WEISS, Mr. WILSON, Mr. WOLF, Mr. WOLPE, Mr. YATRON, and Mr. YOUNG of Alaska) introduced the following joint resolution; which was referred to the Committee on Post Office and Civil Service

AUGUST 1, 1991

Additional sponsors: Mr. BRUCE, Mr. BURTON of Indiana, Mr. CHANDLER, Mr. COBLE, Mr. CONDIT, Mr. COX of Illinois, Mr. DARDEN, Mr. DORNAN of California, Mr. DOWNEY, Mr. DREIER of California, Mr. DURBIN, Mr. GEKAS, Mr. GLICKMAN, Mr. FLAKE, Mr. HOAGLAND, Mr. HOYER, Mr. HUCKABY, Mr. HUGHES, Mr. HUTTO, Mr. JEFFERSON, Mr. KANJORSKI, Ms. KAPTUR, Mr. KENNEDY, Mr. KOPETSKI, Mr. LOWERY of California, Mr. MOODY, Mr. MORAN, Mr. MORRISON, Mr. NICHOLS, Mr. RAHALL, Mr. SABO, Mr. SHARP, Mr. SHAYS, Mr. SIKORSKI, Mr. SKELTON, Mr. SMITH of Iowa, Mr. STALLINGS, Mr. STOKES, Mr. TAYLOR of Mississippi, Mr. TORRES, Mr. TOWNS, Mr. WHEAT, Mr. FORD of Tennessee, Mr. FOGLIETTA, Mr. NAGLE, Ms. SLAUGHTER of New York, Mrs. MINK, Mr. LAROCCO, Ms. WATERS, Mrs. COLLINS of Illinois, Mr. SWIFT, Mr. SYNAR, Mr. LEHMAN of California, Mr. WYDEN, Mr. BACCHUS, Mr. RIT-TER, Mr. DINGELL, Mr. SAWYER, Mr. HOUGHTON, Ms. DELAURO, Mr. SANDERS, Mr. ROSE, Mr. SKAGGS, Mr. BOUCHER, Mr. ANDERSON, Mr. ANDREWS of Texas, Mr. ANNUNZIO, Mr. ANTHONY, Mr. ATKINS, Mr. BALLENGER, Mr. BEILENSON, Mr. BREWSTER, Mr. BRYANT, Mr. COLE-MAN of Texas, Mr. DELAY, Mr. DONNELLY, Mr. DORGAN of North Da-kota, Mr. EDWARDS of Texas, Mr. ENGEL, Mr. EVANS, Mr. FEIGHAN, Mr. FIELDS, Mr. FRANK of Massachusetts, Mr. GIBBONS, Mr. HAMIL-TON, Mr. HYDE, Mr. INHOFE, Mr. JENKINS, Mr. MILLER of California, Mr. MINETA, Mr. MONTGOMERY, Mr. ORTIZ, Mr. PARKER, Mr. PERKINS, Mr. PICKLE, Mr. RICHARDSON, Mr. RIDGE, Mr. SOLARZ, Mr. TRAXLER, Mr. WASHINGTON, and Mr. WISE

AUGUST 1, 1991

Committee on Post Office and Civil Service discharged; considered and passed

JOINT RESOLUTION

Designating August 29, 1991, as "National Sarcoidosis Awareness Day".

Whereas sarcoidosis is a systemic disease of unknown causes that can affect any part of the body;

Whereas sarcoidosis affects between 20 and 50 individuals in 100,000 in the United States;

Whereas most victims of the disease range in age between 20 and 40 years, with blacks being affected at least 10 times more often than other ethnic groups in the United States;

Whereas between 10 to 20 percent of individuals stricken with sarcoidosis eventually develop serious disabling conditions caused by damage to vital organs, such as lungs, heart, and central nervous system;

Whereas sarcoidosis is an enigma in the realm of medicine and disease that requires extensive and ongoing study and research in an effort to develop an effective treatment and eventually a cure;

Whereas individuals with sarcoidosis and family members across the United States are seeking treatment and support services to assist in controlling the effects of the disease;

Whereas grassroot support groups and nonprofit organizations are forming across the United States to encourage public awareness of the mysterious and debilitating disease;

Whereas the Federal Government has a responsibility to lead a nationwide effort to find a cure for the disabling disease; and

Whereas the Federal Government should make research into the causes of the life-threatening ailment a greater priority and provide the public with more information about potential treatments for individuals with sarcoidosis: Now, therefore, be it

1   *Resolved by the Senate and House of Representatives*

2   *of the United States of America in Congress assembled,*

3   That August 29, 1991, is designated as "National Sar-

4   coidosis Awareness Day", and the President is authorized

5   and requested to issue a proclamation calling upon the

1 people of the United States to observe the week with ap-
2 propriate ceremonies and activities.

O

State of New York
Legislative Resolution

Senate No. 481

BY: Senators Levy, Babbush, Bruno, Connor, Cook, Daly, Farley, Galiber, Gold, Halperin, Hannon, Hoffmann, Holland, Johnson, Korman, Kuhl, Lack, Larkin, LaValle, Leichter, Libous, Maltese, Marchi, Markowitz, Masiello, McHugh, Mega, Mendez, Montgomery, Ohrenstein, Onorato, Oppenheimer, Paterson, Quattrociocchi, Saland, Sears, Seward, Skelos, Spano, Stachowski, Stafford, Trunzo, Tully, Velella, Volker, Waldon and Weinstein

MEMORIALIZING Governor Mario M. Cuomo to proclaim August 29, 1992, as "New York State Sarcoidosis Awareness Day"

WHEREAS, It is the intent of this Legislative Body to memorialize the Honorable Mario M. Cuomo, Governor, to proclaim August 29, 1992 as "New York State Sarcoidosis Awareness Day," in coordination with the "National Sarcoidosis Awareness Day"; designated August 29, 1992; and

WHEREAS, Sarcoidosis is a non-contagious, systemic disease of unknown origin and is commonly diagnosed with the detection of inflamed, microscopic growths, called granulomas, which most commonly affect the lungs but can affect any organ of the body; and

WHEREAS, Researchers believe Sarcoidosis results from the inhalation of an infectious or allergic substance from the environment, while others believe it is caused by an alteration of the body's cellular immune system; and

WHEREAS, Sarcoidosis is found throughout the world and affects between 10 and 40 individuals in 100,000; thereby affecting between 1,800 and 7,200 New Yorkers; and

WHEREAS, Sarcoidosis' symptoms can make the disease difficult to diagnose because "victims" do not always have alerting signs; thereby making the impact of this disease on society difficult to assess; and

WHEREAS, Sarcoidosis is most common in young people between the ages of 20 and 40 years. with Caucasians of European descent, Black Americans and Women being affected more often than other groups; and

WHEREAS, Between 10 to 20 percent of individuals stricken with sarcoidosis eventually develop serious disabling conditions caused by damage to vital organs, such as lungs, heart, brain, kidneys and central nervous system; and

WHEREAS, Others afflicted with this disease do not require treatment and improve spontaneously with a self-limiting course of action; and

WHEREAS, Sarcoidosis is an enigma in the realm of medicine and disease that requires extensive and ongoing study and research in an effort to develop an effective treatment and eventually a cure; and

WHEREAS, Sarcoidosis patients and their family members across New York State and the United States are seeking treatment and support services to assist in controlling the effects of the disease; and

WHEREAS, Grassroots support groups and nonprofit organizations are forming across New York State and the United States to encourage public awareness of this mysterious and debilitating disease; and

WHEREAS, It is the sense of this Legislative Body that new initiatives must be developed by the State of New York as part of an intensified effort to educate the public of this dread disease and in support of research into its cause and treatment; and

WHEREAS, The purpose of declaring "New York State Sarcoidosis Awareness Day" is to increase knowledge and understanding of this disease between "victims," the medical profession and citizens of New York State and to encourage those involved to work together for the edification and emulation of all; now, therefore, be it

RESOLVED, That this Legislative Body pause in its deliberations to memorialize the Honorable Mario M. Cuomo, Governor, to proclaim August 29, 1992 as "New York State Sarcoidosis Awareness Day"; and be it further

RESOLVED, That a copy of this Resolution, suitably engrossed, be transmitted to the Honorable Mario M. Cuomo, Governor of the State of New York.

ADOPTED IN SENATE ON
February 25, 1992

By order of the Senate,

Stephen F. Sloan

Stephen F. Sloan, *Secretary*

OFFICE OF THE MAYOR
THE CITY OF EAST ORANGE, NEW JERSEY

CARDELL COOPER
MAYOR

PROCLAMATION

WHEREAS,   Sarcoidosis is a multi-systemic disease, whose
victims usually range in age between 20 and 40
years, with African-Americans being affected at
least 10 times more often than any other ethnic
group in the United States; and

WHEREAS,   Sarcoidosis may affect any part of the body and
symptoms include a dry cough, shortness of breath
mild chest pains, fatigue, weakness and weight loss
and may result in serious disabling conditions
caused by damage to the lungs, heart and central
nervous system; and

WHEREAS,   Because the exact origin of Sarcoidosis is unknown,
the disease remains an enigma in the realm of
medical science and requires extensive and ongoing
study and research in order to develop an effective
treatment and eventually a cure;

WHEREAS,   Since 1982, the Sarcoidosis Family Aid and Research
Foundation, Incorporated, has provided social
support to the patients and their families as well
as developing an ongoing campaign to promote
increased awareness and medical research into this
debilitating disease,

NOW, THERFORE, I, CARDELL COOPER, Mayor of the City
of East Orange, New Jersey, do hereby proclaim
August 29, 1991 as

"SARCOIDOSIS AWARENESS DAY"

in the City and applaud the efforts of the
Sarcoidosis Family Aid and Research Foundation,
Incorporated for its commitment and dedication
encourage all citizens in East Orange to become
aware of this mysterious disease and support the
research efforts underway to find a cure.

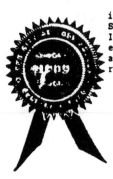

Presented this 29th
Day of August, 1991

CARDELL COOPER

National Sarcoidosis Awareness Day

Jim Slattery
Congressman

I chose to introduce this resolution because I believe that attention should be called to this little known disease. The designation of August 29, 1991, as National Sarcoidosis Awareness Day, has special significance in my office. It is the birthday of my receptionist, Carolyn Anderson, who was diagnosed 5 years ago with Sarcoidosis only after many failed attempts at finding the source of her illness.

There are hundreds of Americans suffering every day from symptoms associated with Sarcoidosis These individuals deserve special recognition for the courageous battles they wage against this disease. By designating August 29, 1991, as National Sarcoidosis Awareness Day, I hoped to focus national attention on the urgent need for continuing research into the detection and treatment of this mysterious and potentially fatal disease. Perhaps more importantly, this national day of recognition gave us the opportunity to provide information about Sarcoidosis to at-risk populations.

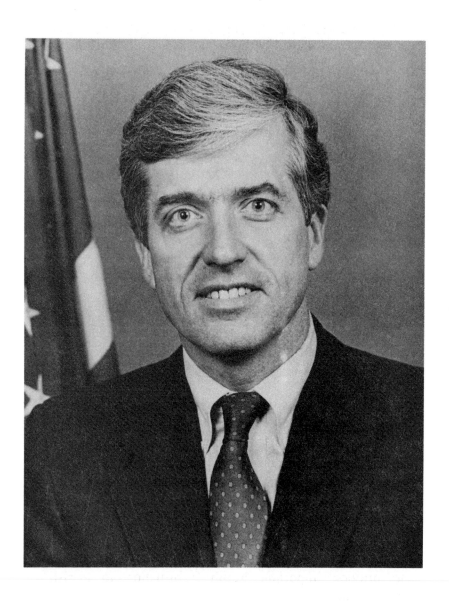

The Campaign Against Sarcoidosis

Kweisi Mfume
Congressman

As will be the case with many readers of this book, I came to learn about sarcoidosis through a friend who had contracted the disease. Like many sufferers, she experienced painful and worrisome symptoms for an extended period, and was run through numerous tests, diagnoses, and treatments before she and her doctors learned she was suffering from sarcoidosis.

My friend's physical and psychological suffering was prolonged because she and her doctors failed to recognize the symptoms, and that delayed proper diagnosis and treatment. When I began to understand how widespread this disease was, and how little the public and even the medical profession knew about it, I realized, like many others, that something had to be done, and that I was in a position to help.

Working with national organizations like the American Lung Association and the Sarcoidosis Family Aid and Research Foundation, and with the support of important national health leaders like Health and Human Services Secretary Louis Sullivan, we have initiated a nationwide campaign to increase public awareness of this disease and to provide important health information to at-risk populations.

In 1990, as part of this campaign, Congressman Jim Slattery (D-Ks) and I introduced House Joint Resolution 519 designating April 16 as Sarcoidosis Awareness Day. We have reintroduced the Resolution in 1991, and we will continue in future years to use this resolution as a vehicle to focus public attention on this disease and help pave the way for fund-raising efforts in both public and private sectors.

Beyond this initiative, I have supported other health-related legislation that will assist research efforts. Because sarcoidosis strikes African Americans 10 to 17 times more frequently than white Americans, and women more often than men, the cause of research and treatment will be advanced by a provision in "The National Institutes of Health Reauthorization Bill of 1991" that requires that women and minorities be included as subjects in federally funded research projects.

The campaign against Sarcoidosis in many respects is just a beginning. I will join others in continuing to sponsor and support legislation that will address Sarcoidosis, and we will continue to write and speak about it. We will do it for love of friends who have been stricken without warning or understanding, and we will do it for those still to contract this disease-that they may face early diagnosis, better treatment, and quicker recovery.

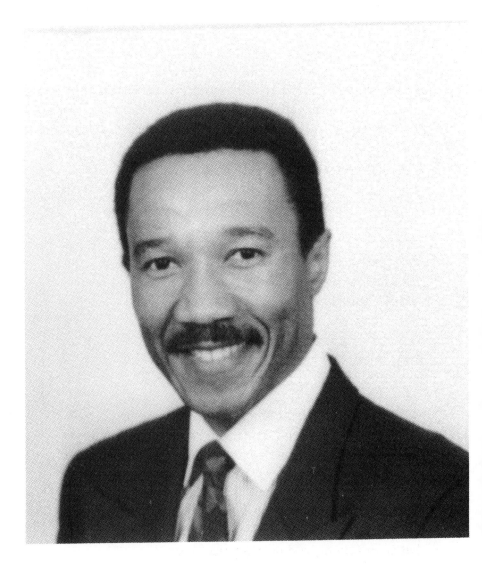

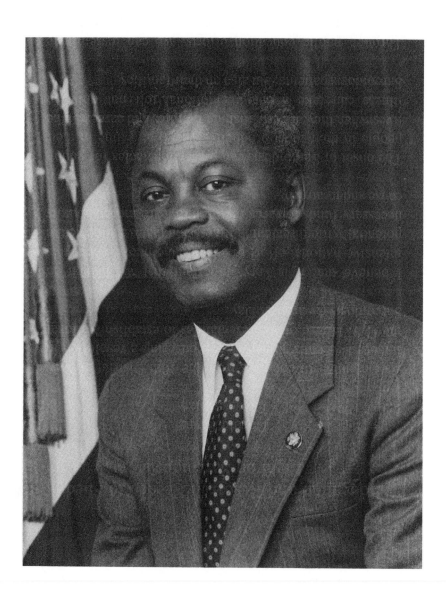

Education and Research Needed to Shed Light on Sarcoidosis

Donald Payne
Congressman

As a member of congress from the 10th District of New Jersey, I recently joined in cosponsoring a resolution in the U.S. House of Representatives to establish National Sarcoidosis Awareness Day.

I believe that it is very important that we launch an intensive national effort to educate the public about this potentially life threatening illness and that we allocate the necessary funds towards research to learn more about its cause and treatment.

The onset of Sarcoidosis can present obstacles for young people in their most productive years, at a time in their lives when they are establishing families and careers. The illness can take a heavy emotional toll not only on Sarcoidosis patients, but also on their families.

Through public education efforts, we can disseminate valuable information about Sarcoidosis to help reduce fear and misunderstanding and to urge those with symptoms of the disease seek medical help.

In my role as a federal representative, I will be working to see that more research dollars are allocated for the study of Sarcoidosis so that we can find the most effective way to diagnose and treat the illness. I look forward to working with the National Sarcoidosis Family Aid and Research Foundation to meet the challenge ahead.

Living with Sarcoidosis

This section of the book has been devoted especially for you. A good idea is to keep a record of your symptoms. Sometimes you might have problems that seem so insignificant or subtle but you should log them down. Keeping records will help you to keep your doctor informed, and should you have to apply for social security disability benefits, you will not overlook any possible medical problems.

There are still many misconceptions associated with Sarcoidosis. The disease itself and it's many different symptoms are often misunderstood. For this reason I decided to include personal experiences from sarcoid patients. You will be able to share their experiences and know that you are not alone.

Also, if you would publicly like to share your experiences with other readers, please mail correspondence to PC Publications, P.O. Box 1593, Piscataway, N.J. 08855.

Please indicate your willingness to allow us to use your words in print.

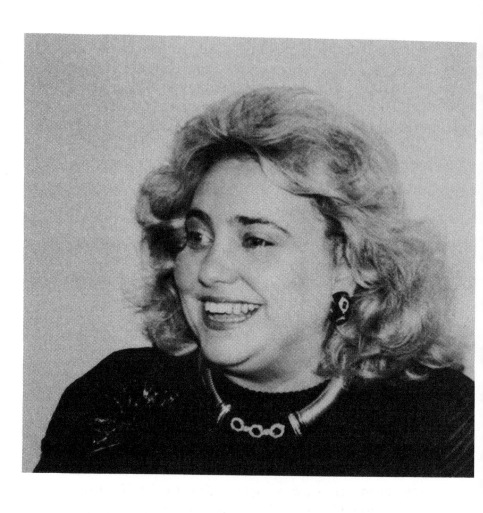

Della Emanuel

Illness strikes like a thief in the night. I had a promising career and felt I was gradually moving upward. I had worked very hard toward a good education and earned a Bachelor of Science Degree in Elementary Education and a Masters as a Reading Specialist. I went on to earn certification in Elementary Administration and Guidance and Counseling. I was an active, well adjusted person and always ready to help anyone. I guess you would say I was the responsible person everyone depended upon. I had an enjoyable social life and shared many good times with close friends. I enjoyed life. I was able to handle any problem area or tragedy. Many had hit our family throughout the years, but I remained strong and high spirited.

I went to bed one evening in 1980 and the thief in the night struck with a vengeance. It would not be till November of 1985 that I found out the thief's name Sarcoidosis. I woke up that morning in 1980 to blurry vision. I had yearly bouts with conjunctivitis, so I really gave it no thought. I used medication my ophthalmologist had given me, knowing it would feel better in a day or so. Only to my surprise it didn't. My vision remained blurred and I was starting to feel various symptoms that were baffling to me as well as bothersome. Every joint in my body ached. I felt like they were doing surgery on my joints and I was awake for it. I had a constant nonproductive cough.

My chest ached and I had difficulty breathing. Climbing the steps was a real chore. I was extremely exhausted and fatigued most of the time. I also had a buccal mass inside the right check of my mouth. I begged for a biopsy of the mass inside of my check. My doctor said it was only a fatty tissue and not to worry about it. I was basically told that my health was due to a classic case of nerves, weight and hypochondria. One doctor told me, I was an over achiever due to my educational degrees in Education. He said, "Stop going to college, get married and have babies." I told him, I loved college. He said, " you think you do, but you really do not and this is your minds way of telling you through the various symptoms your body is feeling." I was not a nervous person, but I was becoming very anxiety ridden. I knew something was wrong with me, but I could not get a doctor to believe me.

The symptoms became worse and I was always at my doctor's office. I finally felt two large lumps under my throat on each side. I felt finally, I had some type of proof I was ill. My doctor put me on antibiotics and told me I had swollen glands. This went on for months and I never got better. Finally a friend who was a nurse, told me to see a surgeon that she felt was very competent. I thought I might as well see him, what did I have to lose after all these years going from one doctor to another. After an examination, he informed me that my lymph nodes were swollen. He recommended I see an ear, nose and throat specialist in Pittsburgh, Pennsylvania. I believe that was on a Friday and I was in Pittsburgh on a Monday. I might add the only other doctor that believed me from the very beginning was my eye doctor.

Suspecting in my own mind I had some type of cancer or Hodgkin's disease I made the trip to Pittsburgh. I was operated on that Thursday. My two lymph nodes were removed, my saliva gland was repaired and the mass inside my mouth on my cheek was also removed and biopsy. I waited for the pathology report to return. I was diagnosed as having Sarcoidosis. I had never heard of that strange sounding word. I guess I always felt if it did not say cancer or malignant it could not possibly be so bad. This is so untrue. This disease runs the gamut from so mild you do not even know you have a problem to chronic, severe and potentially fatal.

I was however relieved to know these painful and distressing symptoms had a name. I can deal with what I know. I was also happy to know I was not crazy as I was made to feel by so many doctors.

I was then sent to a Thoracic Specialist as a chest X-ray had been taken and it was in my lungs. I continue to see him to this day.

I became very ill in March of 1986. I could not walk or talk, and experienced severe problems breathing. I coughed so badly I could not keep my head up. I was hospitalized in Pittsburgh and my Thoracic doctor placed me on Prednisone. It was like a miracle drug. I was so ill, I felt I would surely die that day. The Prednisone worked quickly and I started feeling half way normal, however the side effects were not always pleasant. I continue to take Prednisone, but it is only 5mg every other day unless I get bad.

Sarcoid not only effect the sufferer, but the family as well. I can take the disease, but it hurts when I see the pain in my mother's eyes. I try to be brave and keep my spirits up, but at times I become angry and depressed. We both know I am not the person I used to be. I teach school all day, come home, take a bath, eat, and go to bed. I am completely exhausted by the end of the day and usually in bed by eight o'clock. Sometime I look in the mirror and I am not sure I recognize the image. I look at pictures of myself when I was well and it saddens my heart in a strange sort of way.

I often feel like I am beating out one brush fire after another. Since the disease invaded my body without my permission, I have to let it know it is not welcome and fight it all the way. I started a local support group called

U. S. (Understanding Sarcoidosis) it helps to meet, discuss and offer support.

I wrote to every Talk Show Host in order to get some national recognition and knowledgeable information to the public. I really had to laugh after receiving one rejection letter after another. All were in agreement, the topic was worthy, but not at this time. Upon receiving one letter in particular, I tuned that Talk Show on to hear the worthy topic they were discussing - Why men like to wear their wives clothes! Perhaps I will have to marry someone who wants to wear my clothes, then I will get on a talk show and can sneak in Sarcoidosis!

I have always said that unless someone famous gets this disease no one will know about it. The increased awareness of AIDS came about due to Rock Hudson's death. Elizabeth Taylor's work toward the advancement and funding has helped enormously. Unfortunately, she is not here to fight for those of us with Sarcoid; so it is up to all of us to spread the word and pray someone will listen.

I am not pleased as punch that I have this disease and I would love to go back to the person I used to be. There is no time for bitterness. You have to get past it and fight in a positive manner.

Many doctors are not trained to look for the rare disease. When they do not know what it is, they blame it on weight, nerves or stress. I hope to encourage doctors to dig deeper and most of all believe their patients and listen clearly. I also hope to soften the hearts of our government officials and make them see the need for finances to secure the very much needed research into this distressing and complex disease. We must strive to find a common thread that ties us together.

I write to people all over the United States and we do have one thing in common - the courage and the ability to keep on going and our earnest prayers for a cure.

Matthew L. Robinson

1959 was my first experience with the symptoms of Sarcoidosis. I was nineteen years old, serving in the United States Army. I was stationed in San Antonio, Texas. While showering, my fellow army buddies informed me that I had a scaly rash on the upper part of my back in the shoulder area. I went on "Sick Call" and after examination and scrapings of the rash were taken, I was told that I was probably taking too many showers and my treatment was body lotion and fewer showers.

For many years after my discharge from the military, the rash would reappear. It did not itch or irritate me, but would appear as a puffy circular area with a bumpy looking appearance around the edges and indentation in the middle. It would disappear as mysteriously as it would appear. I went to the Veterans' Hospital, and after examination, was told that they did not know what it was and sent me on my way.

In 1977, some eighteen years later and after the rash had disappeared, I was awakened one Sunday night from my sleep with an excruciating headache. When I made my way into the bathroom and turned on the light, my eyes were blood red and extremely sensitive to light. Aspirins would not relieve my headache or discomfort. When morning came I went to the Ear, Eye, Nose and Throat Clinic at the Maryland General Hospital. The doctor immediately told me, upon examination of my eyes, "You have Sarcoidosis." I was referred to the Pulmonary Clinic.

Upon further examination and X-rays, I was told that my lungs were seriously infected with the disease and possibly with tuberculosis, as well. I was started on anti-tubercular drugs and was allergic to every one of them. I became very ill and one drug caused my entire body to shed skin. The drug was discontinued and I tested negative for tuberculosis.

From 1977 to the present I have been hospitalized many times for various Sarcoidosis-related reasons.

I was hospitalized once because I became very ill with chills, night sweats, fever and difficulty swallowing. I lost about twenty pounds in a matter of a few days and was finally rushed to the hospital when my skin turned dark. I was told that a nodule had grown in my esophagus which had to be removed immediately, because it was causing difficulty in my swallowing. A biopsy was taken at that time, which further verified that I had Sarcoidosis. I was hospitalized for nine days.

Over the years, I have experienced severe pain and discomfort in my chest area. I would get very hot in my chest and have severe coughing spells. My energy left me and I even had difficulty getting up and putting on my clothes in the morning. I would tire out before my workday would end.

I was employed by the prison system and had to be reassigned from my job as a traveling Hearing Officer (Judge) to a stationary job, as Assistant to the Warden of Maryland's Reception Center.

I became very ill before starting my new job assignment and I became bed ridden with severe weakness and pain. The pain in my chest was so devastating, that I would have spasms every few minutes. I could not get out of bed and lost more weight (I never weighed over 135lbs. anyway).

As a last resort, my doctor started me on Prednisone (60 mgs.). I was so weak I had to send out for the medication. When I took the first pills, by morning, I was recovered and energetic. My pain had stopped and I was full of energy. When I returned to work I had gained over fifty pounds and was then reassigned as the Warden's Assistant.

Later I started having difficulty breathing and chest pains. I was told that the Sarcoidosis had affected my heart and the doctor put me on Nitroglycerin patches and pills. I was later referred to a heart specialist and followed by him.

I was appointed as Unit Manager (Warden) of newly constructed prison facility (The Baltimore City Correctional Center) and was given a "transitional team" to help me set up the new facility. The first day that we were together, I was sent for specialized training in how to set up a new facility, I became ill.

Returning from my training session, I was walking through a shopping mall, when I felt my mouth filling up with "something". I put my handkerchief to my mouth and bright red blood was coming out of my mouth. I ran to the nearest bathroom, I was hemorrhaging and spitting up clots of blood.

Some how I managed to drive myself to the hospital. Upon arrival I was examined and told that I had vomited a pint of blood and had I been laying down and the blood had not come out, I would have died. I was later told that I had holes in both lungs as big as quarters and that my right lung would have to be removed. Several specialists were called in and all declined to operate on me. (The hospital's house surgeon was on vacation). They said my chances of surviving a lung operation at that time was less than fifty percent and I would probably not make it off the table.

I was told to wait until the head surgeon returned for the operation. If I hemorrhaged again an emergency operation would have to be done anyway. I was hospitalized and watched for eleven days. I was discharged for the Christmas holidays and told to return in January for the operation. After being discharged from the hospital, I was constantly checking my sputum for blood. I prayed and decided that I would not return to the hospital for the lung operation, this probably saved my life.

I continued running the new facility in Baltimore City for three years, amidst bouts of pain, discomfort, coughing, and lack of energy. Surprisingly getting good reports for running the facility.

My breath became shorter and I had difficulty walking any distance. I would have to inspect the facility almost daily and even had difficulty walking from one end to the other. I was later transferred to another facility in one of the counties, about a thirty mile drive from home. The facility was smaller with fewer inmates who were on a work-release program. However, I still had difficulty walking from my car to the front door of the facility. By the time I reached my office door, the pain and discomfort was so severe, I would close my door and have to stretch out across the desk.

After running that facility for about two years, I decided after getting ill on my Christmas vacation, that I had enough. When I returned in January of 1987, I applied for Disability Retirement from the State. I was granted the disability retirement in May, 1987

Even though I received retirement from the State of Maryland, I had a much more difficult time receiving benefits from the Social Security Administration. The doctor I was seeing had told me that my condition was so bad (the Sarcoidosis) that I did not have long to live and had encouraged early retirement "to do all the things that would make me happy, since I would not live to be an old man". I was forty-six years old at the time. That same doctor had a prejudice about anyone receiving Social Security Benefits and would not submit my medical records to Social Security.

I was still having problems with my heart and was told by the Heart Specialist that I needed an arteriogram of my heart. My primary physician advised against having this procedure due to the danger to my life. I decided to have the arteriogram, and it was discovered that I did not have a heart problem from Sarcoidosis. The Heart Specialist checked my X-rays and was amazed that I had survived with the condition my lungs was in. He advised me to get another opinion of my health from another doctor, which I did as soon as I was able.

The new doctor was surprised at how I looked and got around. When studying my case and X-rays he said I should have been receiving Social Security Disability Benefits years ago. He filled out my forms and did a deposition for the judge (I was at the third step of the appeal by then) and I was granted the benefits by the judge on the day of the hearing. It took two years to get my Social Security Disability Benefits.

Since retiring, I have started a Sarcoidosis Self-Help Group to help inform others. We now meet every other month. To date I have talked with over four hundred people and have helped them through my group. We are sponsored by the Maryland American Lung Association.

It has been a long hard struggle, but I have made it thus far, by the help of God.

I am now maintained on twenty-five mgs. of Prednisone daily. I do have side effects from the Prednisone. I have been on it for about ten years and it has eaten the substance out of my bones in my rib cage. My bones in my chest became very brittle and when I would cough hard they would break. I was first thought to have cancer of the bones in my chest, but after removal for biopsy of a part of my rib, it was not cancer but the Prednisone caused the weakness in my ribs and the breaking. The damage to my ribs cannot be repaired, but I take 50,000 units of Vitamin D three times a week and high dosages of calcium to strengthen the bones that are not broken yet. I cannot go below 20 mgs. of Prednisone or I suffer with severe bouts of coughing and extreme shortness of breath. I still cough a lot and I am still pudgy from the Prednisone. The Prednisone is such a relief for me that I still take it and will have to worry about the after effects later. It helps me to get through the day.

I try to keep a positive outlook, keep as busy as I can, rest a lot, and pray.

Dolores O'Leary

A little background about myself: I am 52 years old and live with my husband Don, of thirty one years, in Puyallup about thirty miles SE of Seattle. We have two married children and four grandchildren. I am a retired registered nurse and secretary. I am also a card carrying clown, white face, wig and all!

Following our only daughter's wedding in May of 1987, my family doctor referred me to a dermatologist because of a skin rash that had been bothering me for a couple of months. After taking a history and noting that I had also been having eye problems (Iritis) since January, the skin specialist took a biopsy which concurred with his diagnosis Sarcoidosis.

Base-line X-rays and a pulmonary function test revealed no signs of Sarcoidosis in my lungs. My ophthalmologist was treating me with steroid eye drops, the family doctor with steroid creams and the dermatologist with systemic steroids and following a consult in Seattle, with the anti-malaria drug Plaquinil.

In July of '87, I developed my first erythema nodosum nodule and anti-inflammatory therapy was started. My eye problems continued and were "upgraded" to Uveitis and for the next eighteen months my treatment continued with local doctors as described above with systemic steroids reduced and sometimes discontinued for a time, only to be started again and used on an alternate day schedule as the rash and/or eyes responded. A referral to the eye clinic at the University of Washington in February 1989, reaffirmed Sarcoidosis involvement in both eyes and a more aggressive steroid therapy was initiated, injection into the Tenon's Capsule which surrounds the eye, in this case the left eye, as granuloma activity was noted on the retina.

Unusual episodes of uncontrolled motor activity in June of that year hospitalized me for ten days. Negative test results did not rule out Sarcoid as the cause of what were now neurological problems. I had begun to develop a peripheral neuropathy on my back and on my legs. Again, I was referred to the University of Washington Medical Center. And again there were no positive findings from MRI's, EEGs or X-rays and they offered no treatment, returning me to my original physicians.

After a second hospitalization in October of fourteen days, I sought a complete evaluation and third opinion as to my health problems at Virginia Mason Clinic in Seattle in November 1989. I received a comprehensive and supportive medical exam with concurrence of the primary diagnosis. I remain there to the present time, under the care of clinic physicians where team evaluation and coordinated therapy continue.

I still have daily episodes of motor activity and the neuropathy is of the sensory class involving my back, legs, feet, areas of my abdomen, chest, face, arms and hands and is painful with stimulation of any kind. I also have joint pain. Even though there is no conclusive proof, it is assumed that Sarcoidosis is the underlying cause. I use self hypnosis with the supervision of a clinical psychologist to help control the pain with a minimum of medication. I am also monitored frequently with blood tests and examinations because of classic steroid side effects. Maintaining my vision is of primary concern and this determines the aggressiveness of Prednisone therapy.

Because of what was termed neuromuscular complications with the Sarcoidosis, I took a disability retirement in November 1990. I continue to be as active as possible with my family, church, and community, Volunteering my time at a variety of tasks. My hobbies of knitting and crocheting have been incorporated in my physical therapy and I use a simple exercise program featured on our local PBS TV called Sit and Be Fit.

Since finding out about NORD (National Organization Rare Disorders) this past summer, I have become part of a local MS support group which is very helpful. I would really like to be in contact with others who have Sarcoidosis. I feel that it is thru networking we can best support each other, even though we may not have the same type of involvement. I have had the personal motivation in recent years to learn as much as I can about orphan diseases and other chronic disorders close to mine. It seems to me that the progress in research and treatment have often come from the constant networking and sharing of patients and their families with each other and the medical profession.

D'Entress Ratcliff

Sarcoidosis: I remember the first time I heard of this disease, and my first thought was by the time I learn to pronounce it and spell it there will be a cure. This was 15½ years ago, and needless to say, although I have learned to spell sarcoidosis and certainly pronounce it, there is no cure.

Sarcoidosis is an unusual disease, due to the fact it resembles so many other diseases, and I certainly am no exception to the rule.

For me, this roller coaster ride began with a bad cold and a cough, while I was visiting my mother in Casper, Wyoming. The cough became part of my daily life, and finally due to its severity, I was forced to see my mother's doctor. After taking X-rays and examining them, he sent me directly from his office into the hospital.

Initially, it was thought, without further testing, I had Hodgkin's disease with a poor prognosis. I have found this to be true with a lot of people with this disease. Once the doctor there had me stabilized, (I had also developed a blood clot), I decided to fly back to San Diego, California for further testing.

I spent five weeks in the hospital, and after dozens of tests and a lung biopsy, I was told that I had chronic sarcoidosis. I was put on large doses of Prednisone, along with other medications, because the disease had also affected my liver, and I was jaundiced.

Through the years, like everyone else with chronic sarcoidosis, I have found it to be quite an education, and certainly not all good. I compare sarcoidosis with a roller coaster ride, because I'm always so thankful when the worst of whatever period I'm going through at that particular time is over, and things smooth out somewhat.

I have been on Prednisone for nearly the entire time I've had this disease, and I have done relatively well, although I readily admit steroids do have side effects, not all pleasant. In my case, when I was taken off the Prednisone, I developed very serious complications with sarcoidosis, both times nearly costing me my life.

Like so many patients with this disease, it has been progressive. But I have found the support of family, friends and a doctor who will listen, and I might add, give hugs. This has been important to how I've dealt with it.

I deal with the pain by keeping as busy as I can; I write, and to the delight of my family and friends, I cook. We may all one day be overweight, but, in my book, I feel it's better than a pill.

Has it changed my life? Certainly it has, and I've found I have to work around it, not the other way around, but my key is and always will be to have a positive attitude, and believe one day answers will be found, and others won't have to experience what those of us now have. Until that time, I choose to see this disease as I would a glass of water, half full, not half empty, and do my best to give hope to others with this disease, as well as people with other diseases.

Notes

PHYSICIANS ASSOCIATED WITH SARCOIDOSIS

Listed herein are the known physicians who currently treat patients with sarcoidosis. With your help, a more comprehensive list could be compiled. If you know of a physician currently assisting sarcoidosis patients, please see Appendix C - Book Forms, page - 283.

Alabama
Jack D. Fulmer, M.D.
Pulmonary Division
University of Alabama
Birmingham School of Medicine
University Station
Birmingham, Alabama 35294
(205) 934-6224

Alaska
None listed at present time.

Arizona
None listed at present time.

Arkansas
None listed at present time.

California

John Parkinson, M.D.
1900 Pennsylvania Avenue
Fairfield, California 94533
(707) 425-1061

Om P. Sharma , M.D.
University of Southern California
Medical Center
1200 North State Street
Los Angeles, California 90033
(213) 226-7923

Spencer Kalman Koerner, M.D.
Cedar Sinai Medical Center
8700 Beverly Blvd.
Los Angeles, California 90048
(310) 855-5000

Jack Lieberman, M.D.
Veterans Administration Hospital
Sepulveda, Calfornia 91343
(818) 891-2327

Warren Borgguist, M.D.
193 S. Fairview Lane
Sonora, California 95370
(209) 532-6223

California

R. E. Lambert, M.D.
Stanford University Med. Center
Immunology Clinic Room A160
Stanford, California 94305
(415) 723-6661

Colorado

Talmadge E. King, M.D.
Cohen Clinic
National Jewish Center for Immunology
and Respiratory Medicine
Denver, Colorado 80206
(303) 398-1302

Connecticut

Jack Elias, M.D.
Professor of Medicine
Chief, Pulmonary and Critical Care Medicine
Director, Winchester Chest Clinic
Yale University School of Medicine
Yale - New Haven Hospital
333 Cedar Street, LCI-105
New Haven, Connecticut 06510
(203) 785-4163   FAX: (203) 785-3826

Delaware
None listed at present.

District of Columbia

Prashant K. Rohatgi, M.D.
Associate Professor of Medicine
George Washington University
Medical Center and
Associate Chief, Pulmonary Section
Veteran Administration Medical Center
50 Irving Street N.W.
Washington, D.C. 20422
(202) 745-8117

Harold M. Silver, M.D.
1601 Eighteenth Street, N.W.
Washington, D.C. 20009
(202) 667-0134

Octavius D. Polk, Jr., M.D.
Howard University Hospital
2041 Georgia Avenue N.W.
Washington, D.C. 20060
(202) 865-6796

District of Columbia

Robert L. Hackney, Jr., M.D.
Alvin V. Thomas, Jr., M.D.
Sheik N. Hassan, M.D.
Wayne P. Davis, M.D.
Rosco C. Young, Jr., M.D.
Howard University Hospital
2041 Georgia Avenue, N.W.
Washington, D.C. 20060
(202) 865-6796

Henry Yeager, M.D.
Georgetown University Medical School
Washington, D.C. 20057
(202) 687-4913

Florida

Allen Rosen, M.D.
1411 North Flagler Drive
West Palm Beach, Florida 33401
(407) 659-1000

Adam Warner, M.D.
4300 Alton Road
Miami Beach, Florida 33140
(305) 848-3860

Florida

Christopher C. Breeden, M.D., P.A.
A. Rogelio Choy, M.D. FCCP, P.A.
3355 Burns Road Suite 304
Palm Beach Gardens, Florida 33410
(407) 627-3335

Georgia
None listed at present.

Hawaii
None listed at present.

Idaho
None listed at present.

Illinois

Daniel Ray, M.D.
310 Happ Road
Glenview, Illinois 60025
(708) 501-4433

Illinois

Alan Leff, M.D.
University of Chicago Hospital
Pulmonary Medicine Clinic
5841 S. Maryland, Box 98 Room W250
Chicago, Illinois 60637
(312) 955-9555

Indiana
None listed at present.

Iowa

Gary W. Hunninghake, M.D.
Professor and Director
Pulmonary Disease and
Critical Care Medicine Division
University of Iowa Hospitals & Clinics
650 Newton Road, C33, GH
Iowa City, Iowa 52242
(319) 356-4187 FAX: (319) 356-7893

Iowa

David A. Schwartz, M.D., M.P.H.
Assistant Professor and Director
Occupational Medicine Section of
Pulmonary Disease Division
University of Iowa Hospitals & Clinics
650 Newton Road, C33, GH
Iowa City, Iowa 52242
(319) 356-8264 FAX: (319) 356-7893

Robert K. Merchant, M.D.
Assistant Professor of Medicine
Pulmonary Disease Division
University of Iowa Hospitals and Clinics
650 Newton Road, C33, GH
Iowa City, Iowa 52242
(319) 356-8268 FAX: (319) 356-7893

Kansas

Donna Sweet, M.D.
1010 N. Kansas
Wichita, Kansas 67217
(316) 261-2622

Kentucky
None listed at present time.

Louisianna

Thomas Senff, M.D.
1801 Fairfield Ave.
Shreveport, Louisianna 71101
(318) 227-8192

Maine

None listed at present.

Maryland

Carol Johns, M.D.
Pulmonary Division
Director, Sarcoid Clinic
Johns Hopkins Hospital
600 N. Wolf Street
Brady 424
Baltimore, Maryland 21205
(410) 955-3467

Stephen Schonfeld, M.D.
4000 Old Court Road Ste. 203
Baltimore, Maryland 21203
(410) 484-9595

Maryland

Stephen R. Selinger, M.D.
R.H. Morgan Professional Office Bldg.
5601 Loch Raven Blvd. Ste. 512
Baltimore, Maryland 21239
(410) 532-4835

Barney J. Stern, M.D.
Director, Division of Neurology
Sinai Hospital of Baltimore
Baltimore, Maryland 21215
(410) 578-5707

Ronald G. Crystal, M.D.
Pulmonary Branch,
National Heart, Lung, and
Blood Institute, NIH,
Bethesda, Maryland 20892
(410) 496-1597

Massachusetts

Barry L. Fanburg, M.D.
Chief, Pulmonary Division
New England Medical Center Hospitals
NEMC #257
750 Washington Street
Boston, Massachusetts 02111
(617) 956-5871

Michigan

John R. Vydareny, M.D.
1900 Wealthy St. S.E. Ste. 115
Grand Rapids, Michigan 49506
(616) 459-1144

Allan Neiberg, M.D.
Critical Care and
Internal Medicine
901 E. Mount Hope
Lansing, Michigan 48910
(517) 484-4033

Minnesota

Richard A. DeRemee, M.D.
Thoracic Diseases and
Internal Medicine
Mayo Clinic
Rochester, Minnesota 55905
(507) 284-2511

Mississippi

None listed at present time.

Missouri

William Pingleton, M.D.
Pulmonary Medicine
Associates, P.C.
851 N.W. 45th Street #201
Corporate Hills, N.
Gladstone, Missouri 64116
(816) 452-8202

Montana
None listed at present.

Nebraska

Louis Burgher, M.D.
Lon Keim, M.D.
650 N. Dr. Building
4242 Farnam
Omaha, Nebraska 68131
(402) 552-2900

Stephen I. Rennard, M.D.
Pulmonary and Critical Care Medicine
University of Nebraska Medical Center
Omaha, Nebraska 68105
(402) 559-4087

Neveda
None listed at present.

New Hampshire
None listed at present.

New Jersey

Andrew R. Freedman, M.D., F.C.C.P.
Philip Mach, M.D.
Pulmonary and Critical Care Associates, P.A.
Brier Hill At Colonial Oaks
C-3 Brier Hill Court
East Brunswick, New Jersey 08816
(908) 390-0044
(908) 937-8181

David Riley, M.D.
Department of Medicine
UMD of New Jersey
Robert Wood Johnson Medical School
New Brunswick, New Jersey 08903
(908) 235-5172

Monroe Karetzky, M.D.
Michael C. McDonough, M.D.
Newark Beth Israel Medical Center
Dept. of Pulmonary Medicine
201 Lyons Avenue
Newark, New Jersey 07112
(201) 926-7863
(201) 926-7597

New Jersey

Larry Frohman, M.D.
Leonard Bielory, M.D.
Immuno-ophthalmology Laboratory
UMDNJ Doctors Office Center
90 Bergen Street Suites 6162 4700
Newark, New Jersey 07107
(201) 982-2025
(201) 982-2763

Reynard McDonald, M.D.
University Hospital
H Level Room 249
Newark, New Jersey 07103
(201) 456-5672

Steven Faigenbaum, M.D., F.A.C.S.
Ophthalmology & Ophthalmic Surgery
Somerset Medical Commons
201 Union Avenue Bldg. 1 Suite G
Bridgewater, New Jersey 08807
(908) 526-4588

Mark Levey, M.D.
349 Northfield Road
Livingston, New Jersey 07039
(201) 994-0441

New Jersey

John Harman, M.D.
Chief of Pulmonary Medicine
2480 Pennington Road Suite 104
Mercer Professional Center
Trenton, New Jersey 08638
(609) 737-7544

Francis Blackman, M.D.
United Hospital
15 9th Avenue
Newark, New Jersey 07107
(201) 268-8087

Arthur G. Pacia, M.D.
445 White Horse Avenue
Trenton, New Jersey 08610
(609) 585-0300

Robert Glass, M.D.
317 Cleveland Avenue
Highland Park, New Jersey 08904
(908) 828-5190

New Jersey

Keith Goldstein, M.D.
189 Rt 31 Suite 106
Flemington, New Jersey 08822
(908) 788-6462

New Mexico
None listed at present

New York

Alvin S. Teirstein, M.D.
Maria Padilla, M.D.
Lee K. Brown, M.D.
The Mount Sinai Medical Center
One Gustave L. Levy Place
New York, New York 10029
(212) 241-5900

Joseph Reichel, M.D.
Albert Einstein College of Medicine
Internal Medicine - Pulmonary Div.
1825 Eastchester Road
Bronx, New York 10467
(718) 904-2983
(718) 904-3405

New York

Charles Felton, M.D.
Joseph Austin, M.D.
Jean Ford, M.D.
Nanette Alexander-Thomas, M.D
Harlem Hospital
Department of Medicine
506 Lenox Avenue
New York, New York 10037
(212) 939-1000

Robert G. Lahita, M.D., Ph.D.
Associate Professor
Chief of Rheumatology and
Connective Tissue Diseases
St. Lukes - Roosevelt Hospital Center
432 West 58th Street
New York, New York 10019
Tel: (212) 523-6658/59
FAX: (212) 523-7442

Jeffrey Siegal, M.D.
1 Barstow Road
Great Neck, New York 11021
(516) 482-7334

New York

Rodger Boykin, M.D.
Critical Care, Internal Medicine
120-31 Guy R Brewer Boulevard
Jamaica, New York 11434
(718) 949-1900

Walfredo Leon, M.D.
115-10 Queens Boulevard
Forest Hills, New York 11375
(718) 793-0075

Luther Clark, M.D.
State University of New York
Health Science Center at Brooklyn
450 Clarkson Avenue, Box 50
Brooklyn, New York 11203
(718) 270-1000

Joseph Donath, M.D.
108-50 71st Avenue
Forest Hills, New York 11375
(718) 380-1553

New York

Gerald Deas, M.D.
109-07 197th Street
Hollis, New York 11412
(718) 776-0586

Alan Friedman, M.D.
888 Park Avenue & 78th Street
New York, New York 10021
(212) 794-2277

North Carolina

Yash P. Kataria, M.D., F.R.C.P.E., F.C.C.P.
Professor of Medicine
School of Medicine East Carolina University
Greenville, North Carolina 27858
(919) 551-4653

North Dakota
None listed at present.

Ohio

James E. Gadek, M.D.
Pulmonary Division
The Ohio State University Hospitals
Columbus, Ohio 43210
(614) 293-4925

Oklahoma
None listed at present.

Oregon

Marilyn L. Rudin, M.D.
Gregory R. Klick, M.D.
9155 S.W. Barnes Road Suite. 830
Portland, Oregon 97201
(503) 297-3778

Miles J. Edwards, M.D.
3181 Sam Jackson Park Road
Portland, Oregon 97201
(503) 279-7680

Pennsylvania

Harold Israel, M.D.
Herbert Patrick, M.D.
Thomas Jefferson University Hospital
1020 Walnut Street
Philadelphia, Pennsylvania 19107-5587
(202) 667-0134

Murray Sachs, M.D.
Joel H. Weinberg, M.D.
David O. Wilson, M.D.
Medical Thoracic Associates
Aiken Professional Building
532 S. Aiken Avenue
Pittsburgh, Pennsylvania 15232
(412) 621-1200

James H. Dauber, M.D.
Pulmonary Service
Veterans Administration Hospital
University Drive C
Pittsburgh, Pennsylvania 15240
(412) 648-9350

Pennsylvania

Thomas Scott, M.D.
Allegheny Neurological Associates
E. Wing Office Building suite 206
420 E. North Avenue
Pittsburgh, Pennsylvania 15212
Tel: (412)-321-2162 FAX: (412)-321-5073

George Gushue, DO
Embarcation Place, Suite 2
Lord Sterling Road
P.O. Box B
Washington Crossing, Pennsylvania 18977
(215) 493-0435

Rosalie A. Burns, M.D.
The Medical College of Pennsylvania
3300 Henry Avenue
Philadelphia, Pennsylvania 19129
(215) 842-7095

Ronald P. Daniele, M.D.
Hospital of the University of Pennsylvania
3400 Spruce Street
Philadelphia, Pennsylvania 19104
(215) 662-6805

Puerto Rico
None listed at present

Rhode Island
None listed at present

South Carolina

Charles Mullens, M.D.
St. Frances Medical Center
Greenville, South Carolina 29601
(803) 233-8063

South Dakota
None listed at present.

Tennessee

William Marinecheck, M.D.
210 Jackson Avenue
Memphis, Tennessee 38103
(901) 526-2721

Texas

Frank Arnet, M.D.
John Revel, M.D.
University of Texas
P.O. Box 20708
Houston, Texas 77225
(713) 794-5161

Donald Marcus, M.D.
Baylor College of Medicine
Houston, Texas 77030
(713) 798-6015

Utah
None listed at present.

Vermont

Gerald S. Davis, M.D.
Department of Medicine
University of Vermont
College of Medicine
Burlington, Vermont 05405
(802) 656-2182

Virginia

Paul Suratt, M.D.
Box 225, Medical Center
University of Virginia Health Sciences Center
Charlottesville, Virginia 22908
(804) 924-2228

Washington

Richard H. Winterbauer, M.D.
1118 Ninth Avenue
Seattle, Washington 98101
(206) 223-6687

West Virginia
None listed at present.

Wisconsin
None listed at present.

Wyoming
None listed at present.

SARCOIDOSIS SELF-HELP GROUPS

A WORD ABOUT SELF-HELP GROUPS

Please note that the following list is <u>Not All Inclusive.</u> As we are notified we will be updating our list in future editions.

As you can see there is a need to develop more self-help groups. You now have the tools to work with, see Ideas and Considerations for Starting A Self-Help Mutual Aid Group for Sarcoidosis - page 63.

Delaware

Sarcoidosis Support Group
Public Safety Building
4th & Walnut St
Wilmington, De
(302) 655-7258

Facilitator
Beth Yoncha
Meet: once a month
2nd Thursday
Time: 7:00 - 8:30 pm

District of Columbia

Sarcoidosis Support Group
Sponsorship with the
American Lung Assoc. D.C.
475 H Street N.W.
Washington, DC 20001-2617
(202) 682-5864

Facilitator: Jim Chamberlin
Meetings are announced
through mailings.

Illinois

Sarcoidosis Support Group
Let's Breathe
2225 Foster Street
Evanston, IL 60201

Facilitator: Brenda Harris
(708) 328-9410

Maryland

Sarcoidosis Self-Help Group
Sponsored by
American Lung Assoc.of Maryland
Enoch Pratt Library
(Northwood Branch)
4420 Loch Raven Blvd.
at E. Coldspring Lane
Baltimore, Md 21239
(301) 560-2120

Facilitator: Matthew L. Robinson
Meet: 2nd Wednesday each month
Time: 6:30 - 8:00 pm

Michigan

Lawrence R. Davis Foundation, Inc.
918 Cawood
Lansing. Mi 48915
(517) 484-7831

Facilitators: Barbara Davis - George T. Davis Jr.
Spiritual Advisor: Reverend Melvin T. Jones
Meet: 2nd Sunday each month

New Jersey

Sarcoidosis Support Group
United Hospitals Medical Center
15 South 9th Street
Newark, N.J. 07107
(201) 676-7900

Facilitator: Jean Curlin - Miller
Meet : 3rd Saturday each month
Dr. Staggers Office 4th Fl
Time: 1:00 - 3:00 pm

Sarcoidosis Support Group
Mercer Medical Center
446 Bellevue Ave.
Trenton, N. J. 08607
(609) 394-4132

Facilitator: Patricia Nelson
Meet: 3rd Tuesday
every other month
Time: 7:00 pm

New York

Sarcoidosis Self-Help Group
Nassau County Medical Center
Hempstead Turnpike
East Meadow, N. Y. 11554
(516) 483-2666

Facilitator: Robert Schoenfeld
Meet: Auditorium each month
2nd Thursday -Time: 7:00 pm

Pennsylvania

U.S. (Understanding Sarcoidosis)
Sarcoidosis Self-Help Group
New Castle, PA 16105
(412) 652-6080

Facilitator: Della Emanuel
Meetings are announced
through mailings.

Virginia

Sarcoidosis Self-Help Group
Sponsorship with the
American Lung Association
of Northern Virginia
9735 Main Street
Fairfax, Va 22031
(703) 591-4131

Facilitator: Carolyn Thomas
Meet: 1st Tuesday of each month
Alexander Hospital
Dudley Conference Room
4320 Seminary Rd.
Alexandria, Va
Group: Educational/Support

FEDERAL INFORMATION

CENTER

The Federal Information Center is one office that has specially selected and trained its staff to answer your questions or help you find the right person with the answer. If your area is not listed, call (301) 722-9098 or if you prefer to write, mail inquiry to the Federal Information Center, P.O. Box 600, Cumberland, Md 21502. Users of Telecommunications Devices for the Deaf (TDD/TTY) may call toll-free from any point in the United States by dialing (800) 326-2996.

STATES OFFICES
Alabama
Birmingham, Mobile
(800) 366-2998

Alaska
Anchorage
(800) 729-8003

Arizona
Phoenix
(800) 359-3997

Arkansas
Little Rock
(800) 366-2998

California
Los Angeles, San Diego,
San Francisco, Santa Ana
(800) 726-4995 Sacramento **(916) 973-1695**

Colorado
Colorado Springs,
Denver, Pueblo
(800) 359-3997

Connecticut
Hartford, New Haven
(800) 347-1997

Florida
Fort lauderdale,
Jacksonville, Miami,
Orlando, St. Petersburg,
Tampa, West Palm Beach
(800) 347-1997

Georgia
Atlanta
(800) 347-1997

Hawaii
Honolulu
(800) 733-5996

Illinois
Chicago
(800) 366-2998

Indiana
Gary
(800) 366-2998
Indianapolis
(800) 347-1997

Iowa
All Locations
(800) 735-8004

Kansas
All Locations
(800) 735-8004

Kentucky
Louisville
(800) 347-1997

Louisiana
New Orleans
(800) 366-2998

Maryland
Baltimore
(800) 347-1997

Massachusetts
Boston
(800) 347-1997

Michigan
Detroit, Grand Rapids
(800) 347-1997

Minnesota
Minneapolis
(800) 366-2998

Missouri
St. Louis
(800) 366-2998

Nebraska
Omaha
(800) 366-2998

New Jersey
Newark, Trenton
(800) 347-1997

New Mexico
Albuquerque
(800) 359-3997

New York
Albany, Buffalo,
New York, Rochester,
Syracuse
(800) 347-1997

North Carolina
Charlotte
(800) 347-1997

Ohio
Akron, Cincinnati,
Cleveland, Columbus,
Dayton, Toledo
(800) 347-1997

Oklahoma
Oklahoma City, Tulsa
(800) 366-2998

Oregon
Portland
(800) 726-4995

Pennsylvania
Philadelphia, Pittsburgh
(800) 347-1997

Rhode Island
Providence
(800) 347-1997

Texas
Austin, Dallas,
Fort Worth,
Houston,
San Antonio
(800) 366-2998

Utah
Salt Lake City
(800) 359-3997

Virginia
Norfolk,
Richmond,
Roanoke
(800) 347-1997

Washington
Seattle, Tacoma
(800) 726-4995

Wisconsin
Milwaukee
(800) 366-2998

COUNTY OFFICES OF THE HANDICAPPED

These offices are a central source of information about services and programs available to physically and developmentally disabled people to facilitate their full participation in community life.

OFFICES ON AGING

Contact these offices for information on Housing, and Legal issues.

SOCIAL SECURITY ADMINISTRATION
(800) 431-2804

National Organization of Social Security Claimants Representatives will recommend local attorney familiar with Social Security issues.

National Sarcoidosis Resource Center

The National Sarcoidosis Resource Center (NSRC) is a new organization founded by Sandra Conroy. During her years of researching information for the Sarcoidosis Resource Guide and Directory, she became painfully aware of the many inaccuracies surrounding sarcoidosis, the limited information and services available to sarcoid patients and the need for such an organization as the National Sarcoidosis Resource Center.

The purpose of the organization is to provide services for sarcoid patients and their families. NSRC provides literature, physicians referrals, a quarterly newsletter, encourages the formation of self-help groups, networking program, and communications. To advance education and research, the center will provide statistical reports to physicians, health care professionals and government agencies.

National Sarcoidosis Resource Center
P.O. Box 1593
Piscataway, N.J. 08855-1593
(908) 699-0733

DIVISION OF VOCATIONAL REHABILITATION SERVICES

The Division's Primary goal is to make it possible for disabled people to continue working. This would include working from the home as well as outside the home. They provide testing, training, and equipment as necessary to keep someone employed. Medical equipment is also provided if no other services are available.

SCRIPT

SCRIPT stands for Statewide Computerized referral Information Program. This program provides a computer printout of information regarding requests for specific services. The SCRIPT database lists more than 1600 facilities providing approximately 5000 distinct services specifically for people with disabilities. To request a free search, call the toll free number between 9:30 am and 4:30 pm, Monday through Friday. The computer printout will be mailed to you, usually within two days.

N.J. (800) 792-8858 (Voice/TTY)
Outside New Jersey
(609) 292-3745 or (609) 292-0054 TTY.

American Lung Association

The American Lung Association (ALA) has given more than eighty five years of service to the American public. It was founded in 1904 to fight tuberculosis. Today there are approximately one hundred and thirty local and state Lung Associations across the country and in U.S. Territories. Each one works to inform the public about all lung diseases and helps to find answers to the problems of preventing, treating, and curing lung disease.

Each association works with local health departments, community hospitals and other agencies to set up the services needed to find, diagnose, treat, and rehabilitate patients. Lung Associations do not provide the services. Instead, they work with and through other agencies, helping to establish or improve services.

The Lung Associations are basically educational organizations. They carry out public health education and professional education, support medical and social research, and stimulate community action needed to fight lung disease. They work for prevention and control of lung disease patients.

Each Lung Association provides a wide variety of educational materials, including written brochures and audiovisuals. Some materials are for the general public, and others are aimed at special groups: patients, physicians, school students, nurses, medical students, teachers, and public health workers.

The major program areas of the associations include air conservation, smoking, occupational health, lung disease care and education, and school health education.

National Organization for Rare Disorders

The National Organization for Rare Disorders (NORD) has been created by a group of voluntary agencies, medical researchers and individuals concerned about Orphan Diseases and Orphan Drugs. Orphan Diseases are rare, debilitating illnesses which strike small numbers of people. Orphan Drugs are therapies which alleviate symptoms of some rare diseases, but which have not been developed by the pharmaceutical industry because they are unprofitable.

Any disorder affecting fewer than 200,000 people is an "Orphan Disease" because products developed for these illnesses are considered by the pharmaceutical industry as "drugs of little commercial value." The cost of developing a drug in the U.S. today ranges between $50 million and $80 million. To provide incentives for commercial development of Orphan Drugs, Congress enacted the "Orphan Drug Act," which became law on January 4, 1983.

Passage of the Orphan Drug Act, however, does not signify the end of the struggle for people with rare disorders; rather, it represents only the end of the beginning. Recognizing that more than 5000 rare disorders affect more than 20 million Americans, NORD addresses their concerns; people with Orphan Diseases do not suffer less pain and their families do not endure less agony simply because smaller numbers are affected by these illnesses.

NORD's objectives are:

To act as a clearinghouse for information about rare disorders and to network families with similar disorders together for mutual support.

To encourage and promote increased scientific research on the cause, control and ultimate cure of rare disorders.

To accumulate and disseminate information about Orphan Drugs and Devices, making known their availability to patients, physicians and other concerned parties.

To foster communications among rare disease voluntary agencies, government bodies, scientific researchers, industry, academic institutions, and concerned individuals.

To assist in harmonizing and making more efficient the work of voluntary agencies and to offer technical assistance to newly organized support groups.

To educate the general public and medical profession about the existence, diagnosis and treatment of rare disorders.

To represent people with Orphan Diseases who are not otherwise represented by organizations or voluntary agencies.

To focus the attention of government, industry and the scientific community on the needs of people with rare disorders.

ALLIANCE FOR DISABLED

IN ACTION, INC.

The Alliance for Disabled in Action, Inc., ADA, is an independent living resource center which is primarily run by and for individuals with disabilities. The mission of ADA is to improve the quality of life and increase the independence for individuals with disabilities through independent living.

Services:
Independent Living Skills Training, Case Management, Information and Referral, Advocacy, Peer Sharing, Newsletter, Social/Recreational Activities.

There are over 300 Independent Living Resource Centers throughout the United States. For additional information, you may write or call :

Alliance For Disabled in Action
2050 Oak Tree Road
Edison, New Jersey 08820
908-321-1600 Voice/TDD

The National Sarcoidosis Family Aid & Research Foundation

The National Sarcoidosis Family Aid and Research Foundation, Inc. is a nonprofit organization founded in 1982, to stimulate research into sarcoidosis, increase public awareness of the disease, and to provide support services for Sarcoidosis sufferers and their families.

Since their inception, the foundation has provided services to approximately twenty thousand individuals and families, organizations, and churches throughout the country.

The Foundation provides information, referral services, counseling, advocacy, and encourages the development of self-help groups.

For additional information you may write or call:

The National Sarcoidosis Family Aid
and Research Foundation
P.O. Box 22868
Newark, New Jersey 07101
(800) 223-6429

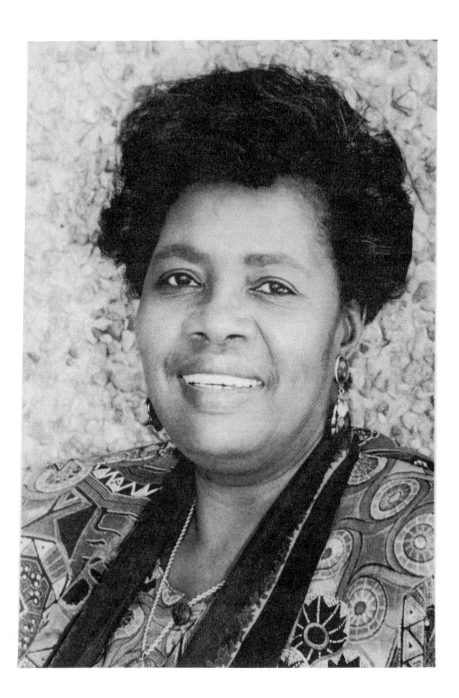

Geneva Ausley

I am very proud to be the founder and president of The National Sarcoidosis Family Aid & Research Foundation, Inc. In spite of the many obstacles that I encountered, with the help of God and the help of a number of concerned citizens, the foundation has helped to increase public awareness of sarcoidosis; stimulate research into its causes/treatment; and provide support services for Sarcoidosis patients and their families.

The foundation was born out of frustration after visiting doctor after doctor with my own daughter who was diagnosed with this illness and finding no appropriate treatment. It was born as a result of a lack of information once the disease had been diagnosed; it was born out of an endless search for resources when medical bills skyrocketed; and it was born when appropriate treatment could not be found. There seemed to be no organization to which Sarcoidosis patients and their families could turn to for support or for a holistic approach to the many problems Sarcoidosis patients faced.

Some of the problems that I was faced with before the Foundation was established included some doctors wanted to get paid up front, the insurance company dropped my daughter's policy and I had to get a lawyer in order to get the bills paid and still ending up with no insurance, struggling to try to keep the family together, trying to run a business, and trying to raise funds. All of this and yet I was still trying to deal with my own personal health problems.

After being treated for years with bronchitis, I was first diagnosed after a growth was taken out of me and tested. It was discovered that I had sarcoidosis instead of bronchitis. My bout with sarcoid was under arrest for several years until I had my house exterminated and then the illness started up again. Once more I had to deal with the general lack of information about this disease.

In spite of the fact that we have been held together mostly by insufficient funding, we are about to celebrate our tenth year of service to the Sarcoidosis patient and their families.

NATIONAL INFORMATION CENTER FOR ORPHAN DRUGS AND RARE DISEASES

"NICODARD"

The National Information Center for Orphan Drugs and Rare Diseases (NICODARD) is an information service sponsored by the Food and Drug Administration's Office of Orphan Products Development. The NICODARD gathers and disseminates information on orphan products and rare diseases to health professionals, patients, and the general public. The NICODARD is a service of the Office of Disease Prevention and Health Promotion (ODPHP) of the U.S. Public Health Service and is operated as a component of the ODPHP National Health Information Center.

ORPHAN PRODUCT An orphan product is one that is used to prevent or treat a rare disease. It can be a drug, biological agent, device, or food. Products to treat rare disorders often get little commercial attention due to the limited potential market. The FDA provides assistance and financial incentives to sponsors undertaking development of these products.

NICODARD answer questions about the source for an orphan product or about clinical trials involving the product. They are generally referred to the product's sponsor. These questions usually come from physicians or hospital pharmacists. Requests for information about a specific rare disorder or patient / family support groups are answered by using the ONHIC's database of over 1,000 health - related organizations. Inquiries are often referred directly to the appropriate organization. The NICODARD does not diagnose illness or provide medical advice. For additional information

write: **NICODARD**
       P.O. Box 1133
       Washington, DC 20013-1133
Call: **1-800-456-3505 (toll-free)**

SELF-HELP CENTERS
AND
CLEARINGHOUSES

For many human problems there are no easy answers or easy cures. Even after the best professional help has been obtained, a person may be left with difficulties too great to handle alone. In this situation, millions of people have found much-needed personal support in mutual-help groups. It is within these groups, whose members share common concerns, that they are offered an important aid to recovery, the understanding and help of others who have gone through similar experiences. Information about self-help groups can be obtained from self-help centers and clearinghouses. Some of these are listed below:

THE NATIONAL MENTAL HEALTH CONSUMERS'
SELF-HELP CLEARINGHOUSE

311 South Juniper St., Room 902
Philadelphia, PA 19107
(215) 735-6367
Provides technical assistance and information and referral services to further the development of consumer-run mental self-help groups.

NATIONAL SELF-HELP CLEARINGHOUSE
GRADUATE SCHOOL & UNIVERSITY CENTER

City University of New York
33 West 42nd St.
New York, N.Y. 10036
(212) 840-1259
Newsletter: Free Brochure

SELF-HELP CLEARINGHOUSE

St. Clares - Riverside Medical Center
Denville, N.J. 07834
(908) 625-7101
Publishes The Self-Help Source Book,
listing 500 national organizations

SELF-HELP CLEARINGHOUSE OF GREATER WASHINGTON AREA

100 North Washington St. Suite 232
Falls Church, Va 22046
(703) 536-4100
Provides information, referral, and support services
to self-help groups in the Greater Washington Area.

SELF-HELP CENTER

1600 Dodge Ave. Suite S-122
Evanston, IL 60201
(312) 328-0470

Publishes in conjunction with the
American Hospital Association
Directory of National Self-Help/
Mutual Aid Resources.

CALIFORNIA SELF-HELP CENTER

405 Hilgard Ave.
Los Angeles, Ca 90024-1563
(213) 825 -1799
California residents: 1-800-222-5465

Publishes Self-Help Group Resources Catalog:
A Guide to Print, Audio, and Visual Materials
and Services for Starting and Maintaining
Self-Help Groups.

Notes

NATIONAL JEWISH CENTER FOR IMMUNOLOGY AND RESPIRATORY MEDICINE

Founded in 1899 by Denver philanthropists to care for an influx of tuberculosis patients, National Jewish is a private nonprofit, non-sectarian medical center. It has become the only center of its kind to focus all its resources on allergic, respiratory, and immune system disorders.

As an international referral center for patient care, National Jewish accepts the most difficult cases from all over the United States and abroad and offers patients the latest treatment methods available.

National Jewish also conducts the largest pediatric allergy and clinical immunology fellowship training program in the world, with 25 percent of all pediatric allergists in America trained there.

RESEARCH

More than $25 million is budgeted each year for immunology and respiratory research. National Jewish researchers publish more than 400 scientific papers annually. Some of the current projects include:

Seeking the genetic trigger that causes lupus, with hope of ultimately eliminating this autoimmune disease.

Identifying immune system factors that can cause allergic reactions. Reaction to food, cold weather, airborne, irritants, and medicine are being studied to provide clues for prevention of severe reactions.

Finding new drug treatments for the growing number of people with antibiotic-resistant tuberculosis.

LUNG LINE

This is a free information service provided to the public by the Center's registered nurses to answer questions about lung and immunologic diseases. Callers can dial toll-free from throughout the U.S. at (800) 222-Lung In Denver, the service can be reached by calling 355-Lung

National Jewish Center For Immunology
And Respiratory Medicine
1400 Jackson St.
Denver, Co. 80206-2762
(303) 398-1002

Bone Clinic

National Jewish Hospital's new outpatient Bone and Growth Clinic aims to help steroid-dependent patients avoid osteoporosis problems while helping victims of the affliction refortify their bones.

The clinic is dedicated to preventing stunted bone growth and reversing osteoporosis (bone thinning), one of the most prevalent side effects of corticosteroids used to treat sarcoidosis and many other diseases. These include, severe asthma, neurological diseases, kidney, liver and bowel disease and rheumatoid arthritis.

Physicians at National Jewish Hospital have closely tracked more than fifteen hundred adult and pediatric patients over the past eight years to monitor steroid effects on bones and growth.

They have successfully treated osteoporosis victims with therapies, including steroid reduction, exercise, fluoride and drug treatments, and diet supplements.

Studies have indicated that only five milligrams of oral steroids a day can reduce bone calcium content and stunt growth. More than fifty percent of all National Jewish referrals who are steroid dependent have medically significant bone thinning or growth retardation. Research has also shown that bone thinning in steroid-dependent patients is worsened by a calcium deficient diet. The clinic uses calcium supplements as one means of increasing bone calcium levels. Exercise is another key treatment. Studies have shown that weight-bearing exercises are effective in maintaining or restoring calcium levels. To detect exact calcium loss due to steroid use, the Bone and Growth Clinic uses advanced bone densitometry equipment to measure osteoporosis severity.

Function of Prednisone in Sarcoidosis

Corticosteroids (**Prednisone**) resemble a substance called cortisone that is produced by the body in the anterior pituitary gland which stimulates the adrenal cortex to produce the hormone. The purpose of Prednisone is to reduce the inflammation of acute granulomas associated with Sarcoidosis.

Nutritional Implications of Prednisone

Potassium Vitamin K+ Hypokalemia

To correct: Adequate intake of fruits, fruit juices, vegetables, vegetable juices, whole grain cereals, meat, and broth.

Sodium Na+ Hypernatremia Water retention

To correct: Eliminate salt - use herbs and spices to season food. Avoid snack foods such as potato chips, pretzels. Avoid processed meats such as bologna, bacon, salami, Canned soups, and vegetables and fast foods.

Protein Metabolism

The administration of large amounts of cortisone may result in a negative nitrogen balance and thus wasting of muscle tissue, thinning of skin, dissolution of vertebral bone, and poor wound healing. Therefore it is important to eat enough protein.

Lipid Metabolism

Steroids increase your total body fat by mechanisms which are still unknown. Fat deposition or "laying down of fat" occurs in specific areas of the body, often in the face, lower cervical vertebrae of the trunk, and the supraclavicular. You cannot change where the fat is deposited because this is a hormonal effect. Research is still scant on the effects of Prednisone and lipid levels such as cholesterol, triglycerides. Studies identify specific groups in which lipid levels are increased while on Prednisone. In theses studies, lipid levels were elevated for short periods of time and returned to normal after Prednisone was discontinued. More research is needed to be conclusive. Lowering your cholesterol intake is a good recommendation for everyone.

Limit egg yolk to 3xs a week. Reduce amount of red meat, use more chicken, fish, turkey. Use margarine instead of butter and use skim milk rather than whole milk.

Carbohydrate Metabolism

Steroid therapy stimulates gluconeogenesis which is the formation of glucose from protein and fat. Persons who are latent diabetics may become hyperglycemic and require glycemia control. Diabetics may require additional insulin. Diabetics should follow at least a "no concentrated sweets" diet and often a prescribed calorie level by your physician or registered dietitian.

Vitamin D

Steroids have an antagonistic effect on vitamin D metabolism so that a negative calcium balance results and osteoporosis may develop. Vitamin D taken daily can prevent this.

Other Effects

Steroids may cause excess hydrochloric acid to be produced in the stomach causing peptic ulcerations which, if severe, could lead to hemorrhage. To alleviate eat smaller meals, and use antacids as indicated.

Mental Reactions

Range from mild irritability, euphoria, nervousness, and insomnia to severe depression or psychosis.

Physical Appearance

Changes in physical appearance occur in most patients on corticosteroid therapy and are emotionally disturbing. These include deposits of fat in the cheeks, upper back, breast, abdomen, buttocks, and thighs, as well as acne, and excessive growth of hair. Most of these side effects are at least partially reversible if doses can be reduced or discontinued.

Ocular

Ocular effects include increased intraocular pressures (sometimes precipitating glaucoma) and the formation of posterior subcapsular cataracts. Regular ophthalmologic examination is advisable.

Myopathy

Muscle weakness and atrophy occur in most patients who receive suppressive doses of corticosteroids for more than a few months. The most prominent involvement is usually in the hip girdle, with weakness on climbing stairs and raising from chairs. Weakness can also occur in the shoulder girdle. If you are experiencing any of these symptoms, talk to your physician.

University of Medicine and Dentistry of New Jersey New Jersey Medical School

Leonard Bielory, M.D.
Director of Allergy and Immunology
Co-Director, Immuno-ophthalmology Service

Interest in evaluation and detection of occult Sarcoidosis, with expertise in systemic therapy of Sarcoidosis, and special interest in the effect of sarcoidosis on the visual system.

Larry Frohman, M.D.
Director of Neuro-ophthalmology
Co-Director, Immuno-ophthalmology Service

Interested in the effects of and the detection and treatment of sarcoidosis involving the visual or neurologic system.

Yale University School of Medicine and Yale - New Haven Hospital

Interstitial and Occupational Lung Disease Program

Co-Directors Jack A. Elias, M.D., L
Lynn T. Tanoue, M.D.

This is a multi-disciplinary program that cares for patients with Sarcoidosis with input from pulmonary physicians, ophthalmologists, immunologists, rheumatologists, hepatologists and when necessary, surgeons. Full diagnostic and consultative services are available. This program interacts with research on Sarcoidosis performed at Yale University School of Medicine.

Personal

Diary

IMPORTANT NUMBERS

DOCTOR:_____

Address:

_____

_____

Phone: _____

HOSPITAL:

_____

Address:

_____

_____

Phone: _____

SUPPORT GROUP:

_____

Address:

_____

_____

Phone: _____

IN CASE OF EMERGENCY:

_____

Address:

_____

_____

Phone: _____

Blood Type:____   **Allergies:**_____
Medication:_____

LOCAL SOCIAL SECURITY OFFICE

Contact Person:

_____

Address:

_____

_____

Phone: _____

LAWYER

Name:

_____

Address:

_____

_____

Phone: _____

Name:

_____

 Address:

_____

_____

Phone: _____

Name:

_____

Address:

_____

_____

Phone: _____

Notes

Date:_____

_____

_____

_____

_____

Date:_____

_____

_____

_____

_____

Date:_____

_____

_____

_____

_____

Date:_____

_____

_____

_____

_____

Date:_____

_____
_____
_____
_____

Date:_____

_____
_____
_____
_____

Date:_____

_____
_____
_____
_____

Date:_____

_____
_____
_____
_____

Date:_____

_____
_____
_____
_____

Date:_____

_____
_____
_____
_____

Date:_____

_____
_____
_____
_____

Date:_____

_____
_____
_____
_____

Date:_____

_____
_____
_____
_____

Date:_____

_____
_____
_____
_____

Date:_____

_____
_____
_____
_____

Date:_____

_____
_____
_____
_____

Date:_____

_____

_____

_____

_____

Date:_____

_____

_____

_____

_____

Date:_____

_____

_____

_____

_____

Date:_____

_____

_____

_____

_____

Date:_____

_____
_____
_____
_____

Date:_____

_____
_____
_____
_____

Date:_____

_____
_____
_____
_____

Date:_____

_____
_____
_____
_____

Date:_____

_____
_____
_____
_____

Date:_____

_____
_____
_____
_____

Date:_____

_____
_____
_____
_____

Date:_____

_____
_____
_____
_____

Date:_____

_____
_____
_____
_____

Date:_____

_____
_____
_____
_____

Date:_____

_____
_____
_____
_____

Date:_____

_____
_____
_____
_____

Appendix A

SARCOIDOSIS

The Early Years

Sarcoidosis

The Early Years

Sir Jonathan Hutchinson-The first descriptions of skin lesions were made by Jonathan Hutchinson. In 1878, the first patient was a man, aged fifty eight. He had a number of peculiar dark patches of dark purplish color on his extremities and he had an attack of gout in the metacarpophalangeal joint of his left forefinger. He eventually died of contracted kidneys. He received treatment at Kings College Hospital in London. Physicians speculated whether the skin lesions and terminal renal disease were interrelated. Mrs. Mortimer, a middle-aged woman, was Hutchinson's second patient in 1898. Her case was so severe, that he called the affliction "Mortimer's Malady" after his patient.

Ernest Besnier-A French dermatologist at l'Hopital Saint-Louis published the first case of lupus pernio in 1889. He described a thirty four year old man with skin lesions on his face and upper limbs. His nose was very large, purplish in color, with a shinning surface. He also had skin lesions on his cheeks. His hands had purplish-red swelling of the fingers. Because of the swellings in the fingers resembling lupus vulgaris (a then common form of skin tuberculosis) and the chilbain-like swelling of his nose, Besnier called the disease lupus pernio.

Cesar Boeck-Was a dermatologist from Christiania (now Oslo), Norway. In 1899 Boeck described sarcoidosis of the skin and lymph nodes. He also recognized that the disease involved more than the skin. In some patients, it involved superficial glands, or mucous membranes (conjunctivae), and in others it caused bronchitis. Boeck was first to understand that the respiratory tract could be involved with sarcoidosis.

Karl Kreibich-Was credited in 1904 for first noting bone involvement in sarcoidosis. In 1921 he accurately described bone changes of the hands and feet in sarcoidosis.

Darier J. Roussy-In 1906 described six women with subcutaneous nodules on the trunk and limbs. Biopsy of the nodules from four of the cases resembled what Boeck had described in the skin. Therefore they called the nodules sarcoidosis.

Heerfordt-A Danish ophthalmologist in 1909 described "febris uveo parotidea subchronica" the syndrome of uveo-parotid fever: uveitis, enlargement of the salivary glands, and cranial nerve palsies. Milkulicz, in 1937, described salivary lacrimal gland involvement in sarcoidosis. It was not recognized until as late as 1937 or 1938 that Heerfordt disease is a form of sarcoidosis.

Jorgen Schaumann-A Swedish dermatologist was chief of the Finsen Institute at St. Gorans Hospital, in Stockholm, Ireland. In 1914 he presented a paper on lupus pernio to the Zambaco Prize Committee of the French Society of Dermatology and Syphilology. His essay was not published until 1934, and for twenty years most of the medical world did not know of his work. Schaumann combined the many diverse syndromes of Sarcoidosis into a single disease.

Lucien-Marie Pautrier-In Strasbourg in 1938 reported the unique pulmonary and lymph node forms of sarcoidosis without skin lesions. In 1945 he reported a natural history of sarcoidosis starting with pulmonary involvement with the eventual appearance of skin lesions.

Sven Lofgren-A pulmonary physician at St. Gorans Hospital in Stockholm and student of Jorgen Schaumann, conducted classical studies of erythema nodosum, febrile arthropathy, and bilateral hilar lymphadenopathy. He inappropriately called this syndrome "bilateral hilar lymphoma," which is known today as Lofgren's syndrome. In 1946 Lofgren studied one hundred and eighty five cases of erythema nodosum and found that fifteen of the cases were probably the results of sarcoidosis. In 1953 a case study of one hundred and thirteen patients, twenty five percent of the patients proved to have Lofgren's syndrome.

Louis E. Siltzbach-New York City, will be remembered as a giant in the research performed on the skin test for Sarcoidosis. Combining his knowledge of clinical medicine, immunology, pathology, and physiology, Siltzbach made one hundred and thirty nine contributions to literature, mostly on sarcoidosis. He also described three radiologic stages of sarcoidosis, and demostrated the effect of corticosteroids in suppressing granuloma formation. In 1960 Siltzbach and his co-worker Merrill Chase reported a new technique for purification and standardization of Kveim test suspensions. In 1966 Siltzbach conducted his famous international Kveim test trail. Thirty seven countries throughout the world participated in this trail test suspension. This survey strengthened the view that sarcoidosis is a single disease entity that is the same worldwide.

John B. Johnson-Founded the Cardiology Division at Howard University Hospital. He was also the president of the American Heart Association. In 1944 in conjunction with Robert S. Jason was among the first to describe sarcoidosis of the heart in a clinicopathologic study.

Claude L. Cowan Sr.-In 1959 confirmed the frequency of eye involvement in sarcoidosis, and described lesser known clinical diagnostic features. He was the chairman of the Ophthalmology Service and president of the National Medical Association.

Harold L. Israel-In 1954, helped established the basis of sarcoidosis as an immunologic disease. In addition to his pioneer work on immunology of sarcoidosis, which he shared with Maurice Sones, he has studied the response of sarcoidosis in patients to BCG vaccination, the interrelationship between sarcoidosis and tuberculosis, and pulmonary aspergilloma in the chronic pulmonary form of sarcoidosis. Israel also worked on the value of gallium scanning in this disease.

Martin Cummings-In 1963, compiled a bibliography on sarcoidosis. It contains three thousand, nine hundred and fifty two references from 1878 thru 1968.

Jack Lieberman-In 1974, described the elevated angiotensin converting enzyme (ACE) in serum of sarcoid patients.

K. Albert Harden-Was the pioneer that stimulated interest in sarcoidosis at Howard University. He was at one time the Dean of the Medical School, head of Pulmonary Medicine and founded the Harden Pulmonary Laboratory. He also was president of the District of Columbia Tuberculosis Association. Harden described the mechanisms in cavitary pulmonary sarcoidosis, and contributed many papers on the many aspects of lung function in sarcoidosis.

LOCAL SOCIAL SECURITY OFFICE

Contact Person:

_____

Address:

_____

_____

Phone: _____

LAWYER

Name:

_____

Address:

_____

_____

Phone: _____

Appendix -B

Index of forms
Part 1

Initial Application

Part 2

Reconsideration

Part 3

Office of the Hearings and Appeals

Part 4

Appeals Council

DISABILITY REPORT

PLEASE PRINT, TYPE, OR WRITE CLEARLY AND ANSWER ALL ITEMS TO THE BEST OF YOUR ABILITY. If you are filing on behalf of someone else, enter his or her name and social security number in the space provided and answer all questions. COMPLETE ANSWERS WILL AID IN PROCESSING THE CLAIM.

. NAME OF CLAIMANT	B. SOCIAL SECURITY NUMBER	C. TELEPHONE NUMBER where you can be reached (include area code)
	___ ___ ___ / ___ ___ / ___ ___ ___ ___	

. WHAT IS YOUR DISABLING CONDITION? *(Briefly explain the injury or illness that stops you from working.)*

PART I — INFORMATION ABOUT YOUR CONDITION

. When did your condition first bother you:	MONTH	DAY	YEAR

A. Did you work after the date shown in item 1?
(If "no", go on to items 3A and 3B.)   ☐ YES   ☐ NO

B. If you did work since the date in item 1, did your condition cause you to change —

Your job or job duties? ....   ☐ YES   ☐ NO

Your hours of work? ....   ☐ YES   ☐ NO

Your attendance? ....   ☐ YES   ☐ NO

Anything else about your work? ....   ☐ YES   ☐ NO

If you answered "no" to all of these, go to items 3A and 3B.)

C. If you answered "yes" to any item in 2B, explain below what the changes in your work circumstances were, the dates they occurred, and how your condition made these changes necessary.

A. When did your condition finally make you stop working?	MONTH	DAY	YEAR

B. Explain how your condition now keeps you from working.

PART II — INFORMATION ABOUT YOUR MEDICAL RECORDS

4. List the name, address and telephone number of the doctor who has the latest medical records about your disabling condition.

If you have **no** doctor check ☐

NAME _____

ADDRESS _____

TELEPHONE NUMBER (include area code) _____

HOW OFTEN DO YOU SEE THIS DOCTOR?	DATE YOU **FIRST** SAW THIS DOCTOR	DATE YOU **LAST** SAW THIS DOCTOR

REASONS FOR VISITS *(show illness or injury for which you had an examination or treatment)*

TYPE OF TREATMENT OR MEDICINES RECEIVED (such as surgery, chemotherapy, radiation, and the medicines you take for your illness or injury, if known. If no treatment or medicines, show "NONE".)

5A. Have you seen any other doctors since your disabling condition began?
If "yes", show the following:

☐ YES   ☐ NO

NAME _____

ADDRESS _____

TELEPHONE NUMBER (include area code) _____

HOW OFTEN DO YOU SEE THIS DOCTOR?	DATE YOU **FIRST** SAW THIS DOCTOR	DATE YOU **LAST** SAW THIS DOCTOR

REASONS FOR VISITS *(show illness or injury for which you had an examination or treatment)*

TYPE OF TREATMENT OR MEDICINES RECEIVED (such as surgery, chemotherapy, radiation, and the medicines you take for your illness or injury, if known. If no treatment or medicines, show "NONE".)

5B. Identify below any other doctor you have seen since your illness or injury began.

NAME _____

ADDRESS _____

TELEPHONE NUMBER (include area code) _____

HOW OFTEN DO YOU SEE THIS DOCTOR?	DATE YOU **FIRST** SAW THIS DOCTOR	DATE YOU **LAST** SAW THIS DOCTOR

REASONS FOR VISITS *(show illness or injury for which you had an examination or treatment.)*

TYPE OF TREATMENT OR MEDICINES RECEIVED (such as surgery, chemotherapy, radiation, and the medicines you take for your illness or injury, if known. If no treatment or medicines, show "NONE".)

Form SSA-3368-BK (1-89)

2

6A. Have you been hospitalized or treated at a clinic for your disabling condition?
If "yes", show the following: ☐ YES ☐ NO

NAME OF HOSPITAL OR CLINIC	ADDRESS

PATIENT OR CLINIC NUMBER

WERE YOU AN INPATIENT? (stayed at least overnight?) ☐ YES ☐ NO (If "yes", show:)		WERE YOU AN OUTPATIENT? ☐ YES ☐ NO (If "yes", show:)
DATES OF ADMISSIONS	DATES OF DISCHARGES	DATES OF VISITS

REASON FOR HOSPITALIZATION OR CLINIC VISITS (show illness or injury for which you had an examination or treatment.)

TYPE OF TREATMENT OR MEDICINES RECEIVED (such as surgery, chemotherapy, radiation, and the medicines you take for your illness or injury, if known. If no treatment or medicines, show "NONE".)

6B. If you have been in other hospital or clinic for your illness or injury, identify it below.

NAME OF HOSPITAL OR CLINIC	ADDRESS

PATIENT OR CLINIC NUMBER

WERE YOU AN INPATIENT? (stayed at least overnight?) ☐ YES ☐ NO (If "yes", show:)		WERE YOU AN OUTPATIENT? ☐ YES ☐ NO (If "yes", show:)
DATES OF ADMISSIONS	DATES OF DISCHARGES	DATES OF VISITS

REASON FOR HOSPITALIZATION OR CLINIC VISITS (show illness or injury for which you had an examination or treatment.)

TYPE OF TREATMENT OR MEDICINES RECEIVED (such as surgery, chemotherapy, radiation, and the medicines you take for your illness or injury, if known. If no treatment or medicines, show "NONE".)

If you have been in other hospitals or clinics for your illness or injury, list the names, addresses, patient or clinic numbers, dates and reasons for hospitalization or clinic visits in Part VI.

7. Have you been seen by other agencies for your disabling condition?
(VA, Workmen's Compensation, Vocational Rehabilitation, Welfare, etc.)
(If "yes," show the following:) ☐ YES ☐ NO

NAME OF AGENCY	ADDRESS

YOUR CLAIM NUMBER

DATE OF VISITS

TYPE OF TREATMENT, EXAMINATION OR MEDICINES RECEIVED (such as surgery, chemotherapy, radiation, and the medicines you take for your illness or injury, if known. If no treatment or medicines, show "NONE".)

If more space is needed, list the other agencies, their addresses, your claim numbers, dates, and treatment received in Part VI.

Form SSA-3368-BK (1-89)

3

8. Have you had any of the following tests in the last year?

TEST	CHECK APPROPRIATE BLOCK OR BLOCKS	IF "YES" SHOW	
		WHERE DONE	WHEN DONE
Electrocardiogram	☐ YES ☐ NO		
Chest X-Ray	☐ YES ☐ NO		
Other X-Ray (name body part here) _____	☐ YES ☐ NO		
Breathing Tests	☐ YES ☐ NO		
Blood Tests	☐ YES ☐ NO		
Other (Specify)	☐ YES ☐ NO		

9. If you have a medicaid card, what is your number (some hospitals and clinics file your records by your medicaid number.)

PART III — INFORMATION ABOUT YOUR ACTIVITIES

10. Has your doctor told you to cut back or limit your activities in any way?　☐ YES　☐ NO
If "yes", give the name of the doctor below and tell what he or she told you about cutting back or limiting your activities.

11. Describe your daily activities in the following areas and state what and how much you do of each and how often you do it:
- **Household maintenance** (including cooking, cleaning, shopping, and odd jobs around the house as well as any other similar activities):

- **Recreational activities and hobbies** (hunting, fishing, bowling, hiking, musical instruments, etc.):

- **Social contacts** (visits with friends, relatives, neighbors):

- **Other** (drive car, motorcycle, ride bus, etc.)

PART IV — INFORMATION ABOUT YOUR EDUCATION

12. What is the highest grade of school that you completed and when?

13. Have you gone to trade or vocational school or had any type of special training? *If "yes", show:*   ☐ YES ☐ NO

    ● The type of trade or vocational school or training:

    ● Approximate dates you attended:

    ● How this schooling or training was used in any work you did:

PART V — INFORMATION ABOUT THE WORK YOU DID

14. List all jobs you have had in the last 15 years before you stopped working, beginning with your usual job. Normally, this will be the kind of work you did the longest. (If you have a 6th grade education or less, AND did only heavy unskilled labor for 35 years or more, list all of the jobs you have had since you began to work. If you need more space, use Part VI.)

JOB TITLE (Be sure to begin with your usual job)	TYPE OF BUSINESS	DATES WORKED (Month and Year)		DAYS PER WEEK	RATE OF PAY (Per hour, day, week, month or year)
		FROM	TO		

15A. Provide the following information for your usual job shown in item 14, line 1.

In your job did you: ● Use machines, tools, or equipment of any kind?   ☐ Yes ☐ No

● Use technical knowledge or skills?   ☐ Yes ☐ No

● Do any writing, complete reports, or perform similar duties?   ☐ Yes ☐ No

● Have supervisory responsibilities?   ☐ Yes ☐ No

15B. Describe your basic duties (explain what you did and how you did it) below. Also, explain all "Yes" answers by giving a FULL DESCRIPTION of: the types of machines, tools, or equipment you used and the exact operation you performed; the technical knowledge or skills involved; the type of writing you did, and the nature of any reports; and the number of people you supervised and the extent of your supervision:

15C. Describe the kind and amount of physical activity this job involved during typical day in terms of:

- **Walking** (circle the number of hours a day spent walking) — 0 1 2 3 4 5 6 7 8

- **Standing** (circle the number of hours a day spent standing) — 0 1 2 3 4 5 6 7 8

- **Sitting** (circle the number of hours a day spent sitting) — 0 1 2 3 4 5 6 7 8

- **Bending** (circle how often a day you had to bend) — Never · Occasionally · Frequently · Constantly

- **Reaching** (circle how often a day you had to reach) — Never · Occasionally · Frequently · Constantly

- **Lifting and Carrying:** Describe below what was lifted, and how far it was carried. Check heaviest weight lifted, and weight frequently lifted and/or carried:

HEAVIEST WEIGHT LIFTED	WEIGHT FREQUENTLY LIFTED/CARRIED
☐ 10 lbs. ☐ 20 lbs. ☐ 50 lbs. ☐ 100 lbs. ☐ Over 100 lbs.	☐ Up to 10 lbs. ☐ Up to 25 lbs. ☐ Up to 50 lbs. ☐ Over 50 lbs.

PART VI — REMARKS

Use this section for additional space to answer any previous questions. Also use this space to give any additional information that you think will be helpful in making a decision in your disability claim, (such as information about other illnesses or injuries not shown in Parts I and II.) Please refer to the previous items by number.

Knowing that anyone making a false statement or representation of a material fact for use in determining a right to payment under the Social Security Act commits a crime punishable under Federal law, I certify that the above statements are true.

NAME (Signature of claimant or person filing on the claimant's behalf)

SIGN HERE ▶   DATE

Witnesses are required ONLY if this statement has been signed by mark (X) above. If signed by mark (X), two witnesses to the signing who know the person making the statement must sign below, giving their full addresses.

1. Signature of Witness	2 Signature of Witness
Address (Number and street, city, state, and ZIP code)	Address (Number and street, city, state, and ZIP code)

NAME OF CLAIMANT	SOCIAL SECURITY NUMBER
	__ __ __ / __ __ / __ __ __ __

16. Check any of the following categories which apply to this case:

PRESUMPTIVE DISABILITY CONSIDERATION
(If any of these boxes are checked, DO's (and DDS's) should be alert to the possibility of a presumptive disability determination in SSI claims per DI 11055.240 and 23535.005.

A. ☐ Amputation of two limbs

B. ☐ Amputation of a leg at the hip

C. ☐ Allegation of total deafness

D. ☐ Allegation of total blindness

E. ☐ Allegation of bed confinement or immobility without a wheelchair, walker, or crutches, allegedly due to a longstanding condition — exclude recent accident and recent surgery.

F. ☐ Allegation of a stroke (cerebral vascular accident) more than 3 months in the past and continued marked difficulty in walking or using a hand or arm.

G. ☐ Allegation of cerebral palsy, muscular dystrophy or muscular atrophy and marked difficulty in walking (e.g., use of braces), speaking or coordination of the hands or arms.

H. ☐ Allegation of diabetes with amputation of a foot.

I. ☐ Allegation of Down's Syndrome (Mongolism).

J. ☐ An applicant filing on behalf of another individual alleges severe mental deficiency for claimant who is at least 7 years of age. The applicant alleges that the individual attends (or attended) a special school, or special classes in school, because of his mental deficiency, or is unable to attend any type of school (or if beyond school age was unable to attend), and requires care and supervision of routine daily activities.

L. ☐ Allegation of Acquired Immune Deficiency Syndrome (AIDS)

17A. Does the claimant speak English? . . . . ☐ Yes ☐ No
If "no," what language does he speak?

17B. Does the claimant need assistance in prosecuting his or her claim? . . . . ☐ Yes ☐ No
If "yes," show name, address, relationship, and telephone number of an interested party willing to assist the claimant.

NAME	ADDRESS	RELATIONSHIP	TELEPHONE NUMBER (area code)

17C. Can the claimant (or his representative) be readily reached by telephone with no communication problems due to language, speech or hearing difficulties? *If "no" DO should complete SSA-3369-F6.*   ☐ Yes ☐ No

18A. Check each item to indicate if any difficulty was observed:

Reading	☐ Yes	☐ No	Using Hands	☐ Yes	☐ No
Writing	☐ Yes	☐ No	Breathing	☐ Yes	☐ No
Answering	☐ Yes	☐ No	Seeing	☐ Yes	☐ No
Hearing	☐ Yes	☐ No	Walking	☐ Yes	☐ No
Sitting	☐ Yes	☐ No			
Understanding	☐ Yes	☐ No	Other (Specify): _____		

18B. If any of the above items were checked "yes," describe the exact difficulty involved:

18C. Describe the claimant fully (e.g., general build, height, weight, behavior, any difficulties that add to or supplement those noted above, etc.):

19. Medical Development — Initiated by District or Branch Office

SOURCE	DATE REQUESTED	DATE(S) OF FOLLOW-UP	CAPABILITY DEVELOPMENT REQUESTED

20. DO or BO curtailed completion of Parts III - V per DI 11005.035 (DI 20501.005)   ☐ YES   ☐ NO

21. Is capability development by the DDS necessary?   ☐ YES   ☐ NO
If "yes", show "DDS capability development needed" in item 11 of the SSA-831-U5

22. Is development of work activity necessary? ....   ☐ YES   ☐ NO
If "yes", is an SSA-820-F4 or SSA-821-F4...   ☐ Pending ☐ In File

23. SSA-3368-BK taken by:
☐ Personal Interview   ☐ Telephone   ☐ Mail

24. Form supplemented: ☐ Yes   ☐ No
If "yes" by:
☐ Personal Interview   ☐ Telephone   ☐ Mail

SIGNATURE OF DO OR BO INTERVIEWER OR REVIEWER	TITLE	DATE

VOCATIONAL REPORT

This report supplements the Disability Report (Form SSA-3368-BK) by requesting additional information about your past work experience. **PLEASE PRINT, TYPE, OR WRITE CLEARLY AND ANSWER ALL ITEMS TO THE BEST OF YOUR ABILITY.** If you are filing on behalf of someone else, enter his or her name and Social Security number in the space provided and answer all questions. COMPLETE ANSWERS WILL AID IN PROCESSING THE CLAIM.

PRIVACY ACT/PAPERWORK REDUCTION ACT NOTICE: The Social Security Administration is authorized to collect the information on this form under sections 205(a), 223(d) and 1633(a) of the Social Security Act. The information on this form is needed by Social Security to make a decision on your claim. While giving us the information on this form is voluntary, failure to provide all or part of the requested information could prevent an accurate or timely decision on your claim and could result in the loss of benefits. Although the information you furnish on this form is almost never used for any purpose other than making a determination on your disability claim, such information may be disclosed by the Social Security Administration as follows: (1) To enable a third party or agency to assist Social Security in establishing rights to Social Security benefits and/or coverage; (2) to comply with Federal laws requiring the release of information from Social Security records (e.g., to the General Accounting Office and the Veterans Administration); and (3) to facilitate statistical research and audit activities necessary to assure the integrity and improvement of the Social Security programs (e.g., to the Bureau of the Census and private concerns under contract to Social Security). These and other reasons why information about you may be used or given out are explained in the _Federal Register_. If you would like more information about this, any Social Security office can assist you.

Public reporting burden for this collection of information is estimated to average 30 minutes per response, including the time for reviewing instructions, searching existing data sources, gathering and maintaining the data needed, and completing and reviewing the collection of information. Send comments regarding this burden estimate or any other aspect of this collection of information, including suggestions for reducing this burden to the Social Security Administration ATTN: Reports Clearance Officer,1-A-21 Operations Bldg., Baltimore, MD 21235 and to the Office of Management and Budget, Paperwork Reduction Project (OMB #0960-0141), Washington, D.C. 20503.

A. Name of Claimant	B. Social Security Number	C. Telephone number where you can be reached (include area code)

PART I — INFORMATION ABOUT YOUR WORK HISTORY

List all jobs you have had in the last 15 years before you stopped working, beginning with your usual job; normally, this will be the kind of work you did the longest. (If you have a 6th grade education or less, **AND** did only heavy unskilled labor for 35 years or more, list all of the jobs you have had since you began to work. If you need more space, use Part III.) If you have already given information about your usual job on the Form SSA-3368-BK (Disability Report), begin with your other jobs.

JOB TITLE (Be sure to begin with your usual job)	TYPE OF BUSINESS	DATES WORKED (Month and Year) FROM	TO	DAYS PER WEEK	RATE OF PAY (Per hour. day. week. month or year)
1					
2					
3					
4					
5					
6					
7					
8					
9					
10					
11					
12					

PART II — INFORMATION ABOUT YOUR JOB DUTIES

Provide the following information (on pages 2-5) for each of the jobs listed in Part I starting with your usual job:

Job Title (from Part I):

A. In your job did you:
- Use machines, tools, or equipment of any kind?   ☐ Yes   ☐ No
- Use technical knowledge or skills?   ☐ Yes   ☐ No
- Do any writing, complete reports, or perform similar duties?   ☐ Yes   ☐ No
- Have supervisory responsibilities?   ☐ Yes   ☐ No

B. Describe your basic duties (explain what you did and how you did it) below. Also, explain all "Yes" answers by giving a FULL DESCRIPTION of: the types of machines, tools, or equipment you used and the exact operation you performed; the technical knowledge or skills involved; the type of writing you did, and the nature of any reports; and the number of people you supervised and the extent of your supervision:

C. Describe the kind and amount of physical activity this job involved during a typical day in terms of:
- **Walking** (circle the number of hours a day spent walking) — 0 1 2 3 4 5 6 7 8
- **Standing** (circle the number of hours a day spent standing) — 0 1 2 3 4 5 6 7 8
- **Sitting** (circle the number of hours a day spent sitting) — 0 1 2 3 4 5 6 7 8
- **Bending** (circle how often a day you had to bend) — Never · Occasionally · Frequently · Constantly
- **Lifting and Carrying:** Describe what was lifted, and how far it was carried. Check below heaviest weight lifted, and weight frequently lifted and/or carried.

Heaviest weight lifted	Weight frequently lifted/carried
☐ 10 lbs.	☐ Up to 10 lbs.
☐ 20 lbs.	☐ Up to 25 lbs.
☐ 50 lbs.	☐ Up to 50 lbs.
☐ 100 lbs.	☐ Over 50 lbs.
☐ Over 100 lbs.	

Form SSA-3369-F6 (1-89)   2

Job Title (from Part I): _____

A. In your job did you: • Use machines, tools, or equipment of any kind?   ☐ Yes   ☐ No

                       • Use technical knowledge or skills?   ☐ Yes   ☐ No

                       • Do any writing, complete reports, or perform   ☐ Yes   ☐ No
                          similar duties?

                       • Have supervisory responsibilities?   ☐ Yes   ☐ No

---

B. Describe your basic duties (explain what you did and how you did it) below. Also, explain all "Yes" answers by giving a FULL DESCRIPTION of: the types of machines, tools, or equipment you used and the exact operation you performed; the technical knowledge or skills involved; the type of writing you did, and the nature of any reports; and the number of people you supervised and the extent of your supervision:

C. Describe the kind and amount of physical activity this job involved during a typical day in terms of:

• **Walking** (circle the number of hours a day spent walking) — 0 1 2 3 4 5 6 7 8

• **Standing** (circle the number of hours a day spent standing) — 0 1 2 3 4 5 6 7 8

• **Sitting** (circle the number of hours a day spent sitting) — 0 1 2 3 4 5 6 7 8

• **Bending** (circle how often a day you had to bend) — Never · Occasionally · Frequently · Constantly

• **Lifting and Carrying:** Describe what was lifted, and how far it was carried. Check below heaviest weight lifted, and weight frequently lifted and/or carried.

Heaviest weight lifted	Weight frequently lifted/carried
☐ 10 lbs.	☐ Up to 10 lbs.
☐ 20 lbs.	☐ Up to 25 lbs.
☐ 50 lbs.	☐ Up to 50 lbs.
☐ 100 lbs	☐ Over 50 lbs.
☐ Over 100 lbs.	

Job Title (from Part I):

A. In your job did you:
- Use machines, tools, or equipment of any kind? ☐ Yes ☐ No
- Use technical knowledge or skills? ☐ Yes ☐ No
- Do any writing, complete reports, or perform similar duties? ☐ Yes ☐ No
- Have supervisory responsibilities? ☐ Yes ☐ No

B. Describe your basic duties (explain what you did and how you did it) below. Also, explain all "Yes" answers by giving a FULL DESCRIPTION of: the types of machines, tools, or equipment you used and the exact operation you performed; the technical knowledge or skills involved; the type of writing you did, and the nature of any reports; and the number of people you supervised and the extent of your supervision:

C. Describe the kind and amount of physical activity this job involved during a typical day in terms of:

- **Walking** (circle the number of hours a day spent walking) — 0 1 2 3 4 5 6 7 8
- **Standing** (circle the number of hours a day spent standing) — 0 1 2 3 4 5 6 7 8
- **Sitting** (circle the number of hours a day spent sitting) — 0 1 2 3 4 5 6 7 8
- **Bending** (circle how often a day you had to bend) — Never · Occasionally · Frequently · Constantly
- **Lifting and Carrying:** Describe what was lifted, and how far it was carried. Check below heaviest weight lifted, and weight frequently lifted and/or carried.

Heaviest weight lifted	Weight frequently lifted/carried
☐ 10 lbs.	☐ Up to 10 lbs.
☐ 20 lbs.	☐ Up to 25 lbs.
☐ 50 lbs.	☐ Up to 50 lbs.
☐ 100 lbs.	☐ Over 50 lbs.
☐ Over 100 lbs.	

Form SSA-3369-F6 (1-89)

4

Job Title (from Part I): _____

A. In your job did you:
- Use machines, tools, or equipment of any kind?   ☐ Yes   ☐ No
- Use technical knowledge or skills?   ☐ Yes   ☐ No
- Do any writing, complete reports, or perform similar duties?   ☐ Yes   ☐ No
- Have supervisory responsibilities?   ☐ Yes   ☐ No

B. Describe your basic duties (explain what you did and how you did it) below. Also, explain all "Yes" answers by giving a FULL DESCRIPTION of: the types of machines, tools, or equipment you used and the exact operation you performed; the technical knowledge or skills involved; the type of writing you did, and the nature of any reports; and the number of people you supervised and the extent of your supervision:

C. Describe the kind and amount of physical activity this job involved during a typical day in terms of:

- **Walking** (circle the number of hours a day spent walking) — 0 1 2 3 4 5 6 7 8
- **Standing** (circle the number of hours a day spent standing) — 0 1 2 3 4 5 6 7 8
- **Sitting** (circle the number of hours a day spent sitting) — 0 1 2 3 4 5 6 7 8
- **Bending** (circle how often a day you had to bend) — Never · Occasionally · Frequently Constantly
- **Lifting and Carrying:** Describe what was lifted, and how far it was carried. Check below heaviest weight lifted, and weight frequently lifted and/or carried.

Heaviest weight lifted	Weight frequently lifted/carried
☐ 10 lbs.	☐ Up to 10 lbs.
☐ 20 lbs.	☐ Up to 25 lbs.
☐ 50 lbs.	☐ Up to 50 lbs.
☐ 100 lbs	☐ Over 50 lbs.
☐ Over 100 lbs.	

IF YOU NEED ADDITIONAL SPACE TO PROVIDE INFORMATION ABOUT OTHER JOBS LISTED IN PART I OF THIS FORM, USE PART III OR ASK THE SOCIAL SECURITY OFFICE FOR ADDITIONAL COPIES OF THIS FORM.

Form SSA-3369-F6 (1-89)

5

PART III — REMARKS

Use this section for any other information you may want to give about your work history, or to provide any other remarks you may want to make to support your disability claim:

_____

_____

_____

_____

_____

_____

_____

_____

_____

_____

_____

_____

_____

_____

(If you need more space, use separate sheets of paper.)

Knowing that anyone making a false statement or representation of a material fact for use in determining a right to payment under the Social Security Act commits a crime punishable under Federal law, I certify that the above statements are true.

NAME (Signature of Claimant or Person Filing on the Claimant's Behalf)

SIGN
HERE ▶ _____ DATE _____

Witnesses are required ONLY if this statement has been signed by mark (X) above. If signed by mark (X), two witnesses to the signing who know the person making the statement must sign below, giving their full addresses.

1. Signature of Witness	2. Signature of Witness
Address (Number and street, city, state, and ZIP code)	Address (Number and street, city, state, and ZIP code)

Do not write below this line

SSA-3369-F6 taken by: ☐ PERSONAL INTERVIEW ☐ TELEPHONE ☐ MAIL	FORM SUPPLEMENTED: If "Yes," by ☐ PERSONAL INTERVIEW		☐ YES ☐ NO ☐ TELEPHONE ☐ MAIL
SIGNATURE OF INTERVIEWER OR REVIEWER	TITLE (also check office) ☐ DDS ☐ DO ☐ BO		DATE

DEPARTMENT OF HEALTH AND HUMAN SERVICES
Social Security Administration

[ ] TEL

Form Approved
OMB No. 0960-0060

TOE 120-145

(Do not write in this space)

APPLICATION FOR DISABILITY INSURANCE BENEFITS

I apply for a period of disability and/or all insurance benefits for which I am eligible under title II and part A of title XVIII of the Social Security Act, as presently amended.

PART I—INFORMATION ABOUT THE DISABLED WORKER

1. (a) PRINT your name ———→ FIRST NAME, MIDDLE INITIAL, LAST NAME

   (b) Enter your name at birth if different from item (a) ———→

   (c) Check (√) whether you are ————————————→ ☐ Male ☐ Female

2. Enter your Social Security Number ————————→ __ __ __ / __ __ / __ __ __ __

3. (a) Enter your date of birth ————————————→ MONTH, DAY, YEAR

   (b) Enter name of State or foreign country where your were born. ———→

   If you have already presented, or if you are now presenting, a public or religious record of your birth established before you were age 5, go on to item 4.

   (c) Was a public record of your birth made before you were age 5? ☐ Yes ☐ No ☐ Unknown

   (d) Was a religious record of your birth made before you were age 5? ☐ Yes ☐ No ☐ Unknown

4. (a) What is your disabling condition? (Briefly describe the injury or illness that prevents, or has prevented, you from working.)

   (b) Is your injury or illness related to your work in any way? ———→ ☐ Yes ☐ No

5. (a) When did you become unable to work because of your disabling condition? ———→ MONTH, DAY, YEAR

   (b) Are you still disabled? (If "Yes," go on to item 6.)
   (If "No," answer (c).) ———→ ☐ Yes ☐ No

   (c) If you are no longer disabled, enter the date your disability ended. ———→ MONTH, DAY, YEAR

6. (a) Have you (or has someone on your behalf) ever filed an application for Social Security benefits, a period of disability under Social Security, supplemental security income, or hospital or medical insurance under Medicare? ———→ ☐ Yes (If "Yes," answer (b) and (c).) ☐ No (If "No," or "Unknown" go on to item 7.) ☐ Unknown

   (b) Enter name of person on whose Social Security record you filed other application. ———→

   (c) Enter Social Security Number of person named in (b).
   If unknown, check this block. ☐ ———→ __ __ __ / __ __ / __ __ __ __

7. (a) Were you in the active military or naval service (including Reserve or National Guard active duty or active duty for training) after September 7, 1939 and before 1968? ———→ ☐ Yes (If "Yes," answer (b) and (c).) ☐ No (If "No," go on to item 8.)

   (b) Enter dates of service ———→ FROM: (month, year)   TO: (month, year)

   (c) Have you _ever_ been (or will you be) eligible for a monthly benefit from a military or civilian Federal agency? (include Veterans Administration benefits _only_ if you waived military retirement pay) ———→ ☐ Yes ☐ No

Form SSA-16-F6 (7-89)   Destroy Prior Editions   Page 1

8.	(a) Have you filed (or do your intend to file) for any other public disability benefits? (Include workers' compensation and Black Lung benefits) ➔	☐ Yes (If "Yes," answer (b).)	☐ No (If "No," go on to item 9.)

(b) The other public disability benefit(s) you have filed (or intend to file) for is (Check as many as apply):

☐ Veterans Administration Benefits   ☐ Welfare

☐ Supplemental Security Income   ☐ Other (If "Other," complete a Workers' Compensation/Public Disability Benefit Questionnaire)

9.	(a) Have you ever engaged in work that was covered under the social security system of a country other than the United States? (If "Yes," answer (b).) (If "No," go on to item 10.) ➔	☐ Yes	☐ No

(b) List the country(ies): ➔

10.	(a) Are you entitled to, or do you expect to become entitled to, a pension or annuity based on your work after 1956 not covered by Social Security?	☐ Yes (If "Yes," answer (b) and (c).)	☐ No (If "No," go on to item 11.)

		MONTH	YEAR
(b) ☐ I became entitled, or expect to become entitled, beginning			
(c) ☐ I became eligible, or expect to become eligible, beginning			

I agree to notify the Social Security Administration if I become entitled to a pension or annuity based on my employment after 1956 not covered by Social Security, or if such pension of annuity stops.

11.	(a) Did you have wages or self-employment income covered under Social Security in all years from 1978 through last year?	☐ Yes ☐ No (If "Yes," skip to item 12.) (If "No," answer (b).)

(b) List the years from 1978 through last year in which you did not have wages or self-employment income covered under Social Security.

12. Enter below the names and addresses of all the persons, companies, or Government agencies for whom you have worked this year and last year. IF NONE, WRITE "NONE" BELOW AND GO ON TO ITEM 14.

NAME AND ADDRESS OF EMPLOYER (If you had more than one employer, please list them in order beginning with your last (most recent) employer)	Work Began		Work Ended (If still working show "Not ended")	
	MONTH	YEAR	MONTH	YEAR
(If you need more space, use "Remarks" space on page 4.)				

13.	May the Social Security Administration or the State agency reviewing your case ask your employers for information needed to process your claim?	☐ Yes	☐ No

14. THIS ITEM MUST BE COMPLETED, EVEN IF YOU WERE AN EMPLOYEE.

(a) Were you self-employed this year and last year? (If "Yes," answer (b).) (If "No," go on to item 15.) ➔	☐ Yes	☐ No

(b) Check the year or years in which you were self-employed	In what kind of trade or business were you self-employed? (For example, storekeeper, farmer, physician)	Were your net earnings from your trade or business $400 or more? (Check "Yes" or "No")	
☐ This Year			
☐ Last Year		☐ Yes	☐ No
☐ Year before last		☐ Yes	☐ No

15.	(a) How much were your total earnings last year? (Count both wages and self-employment income. If none, write "None.") ➔	Amount $ _____
	(b) How much have you earned so far this year? (If none, write "None.") ➔	Amount $ _____

Form SSA-16-F6 (7-89)   Page 2

(c) Did you receive any money from an employer(s) on or after the date in item 5(a) when you became unable to work because of your disability? (If "Yes," give amounts and explain in "Remarks" on page 4.) ➞	☐ Yes ☐ No Amount $ _____
(d) Do you expect to receive any additional money from an employer such as sick pay, vacation pay, other special pay? (If "Yes," please give amounts and explain in "Remarks" on page 4.) ➞	☐ Yes ☐ No Amount $ _____

PART II—INFORMATION ABOUT THE DISABLED WORKER AND SPOUSE

16. Have you ever been married? ➞ (If "Yes," answer item 17.) (If "No," go on to item 18.)	☐ Yes ☐ No

17. (a) Give the following information about your current marriage. If not currently married, show your last marriage below.

To whom married		When (Month, day, year)	Where (Name of City and State)
Your current or last marriage	How marriage ended (If still in effect, write "Not ended.")	When (Month, day, year)	Where (Name of City and State)
	Marriage performed by ☐ Clergyman or public official ☐ Other (Explain in Remarks)	Spouse's date of birth (or age)	If spouse deceased, give date of death
	Spouse's Social Security Number (If none or unknown, so indicate) ___ ___ ___ / ___ ___ / ___ ___ ___ ___		

(b) Give the following information about each of your previous marriages. (If none, write "NONE.")

To whom married		When (Month, day, year)	Where (Name of City and State)
Your previous marriage	How marriage ended	When (Month, day, year)	Where (Name of City and State)
	Marriage performed by ☐ Clergyman or public official ☐ Other (Explain in Remarks)	Spouse's date of birth (or age)	If spouse deceased, give date of death
	Spouse's Social Security Number (If none or unknown, so indicate) ___ ___ ___ / ___ ___ / ___ ___ ___ ___		

(Use a separate statement for information about any other marriages.)

18. Have you or your spouse worked in the railroad industry for 7 years or more? ➞	☐ Yes ☐ No

PART III—INFORMATION ABOUT THE DEPENDENTS OF THE DISABLED WORKER

19. If your claim for disability benefits is approved, your children (including natural children, adopted children, and stepchildren) or dependent grandchildren (including stepgrandchildren) may be eligible for benefits based on your earnings record.

List below: FULL NAME OF ALL such children who are now or were in the past 12 months UNMARRIED and:
- UNDER AGE 18
- AGE 18 TO 19 AND ATTENDING SECONDARY SCHOOL
- DISABLED OR HANDICAPPED (age 18 or over and disability began before age 22)

(IF THERE ARE NO SUCH CHILDREN, WRITE "NONE" BELOW AND GO ON TO ITEM 20.)

20. Do you have a dependent parent who was receiving at least one-half support from you when you became unable to work because of your disability? (If "Yes," enter name and address in "Remarks" on page 4.)	☐ Yes ☐ No

IMPORTANT INFORMATION ABOUT DISABILITY INSURANCE BENEFITS —
PLEASE READ CAREFULLY

I. **SUBMITTING MEDICAL EVIDENCE:** I understand that as a claimant for disability benefits, I am responsible for providing medical evidence showing the nature and extent of my disability. I may be asked either to submit the evidence myself or to assist the Social Security Administration in obtaining the evidence. If such evidence is not sufficient to arrive at a determination, I may be requested by the State Disability Determination Service to have an independent examination at the expense of the Social Security Administration.

II. **RELEASE OF INFORMATION:** I authorize any physician, hospital, agency or other organization to disclose to the Social Security Administration, or to the State Agency that may review my claim or continuing disability, any medical record or other information about my disability.

I also authorize the Social Security Administration to release medical information from my records, only as necessary to process my claim, as follows:

- Copies of medical information may be provided to a physician or medical institution prior to my appearance for an independent medical examination if an examination is necessary.
- Results of any such independent examination may be provided to my personal physician.
- Information may be furnished to any contractor for transcription, typing, record copying, or other related clerical or administrative service performed for the State Disability Determination Service.
- The State Vocational Rehabilitation Agency may review any evidence necessary for determining my eligibility for rehabilitative services.

THIS MUST BE ANSWERED ▶ 21. DO YOU UNDERSTAND AND AGREE WITH THE AUTHORIZATIONS GIVEN ABOVE?

☐ Yes ☐ No (If "No," explain why in "Remarks.")

22. Check if applicable:

( ) I am not submitting evidence of the deceased's earnings that are not yet on his/her earnings record. I understand that these earnings will be included automatically within 24 months, and any increase in my benefits will be paid with full retroactivity.

REMARKS (You may use this space for any explanation. If you need more space, attach a separate sheet.)

III. **REPORTING RESPONSIBILITIES:** I agree to promptly notify Social Security if:

- My MEDICAL CONDITION IMPROVES so that I would be able to work, even though I have not yet returned to work.
- I GO TO WORK whether as an employee or a self-employed person.
- I apply for or begin to receive a workers' compensation (including black lung benefits) or another public disability benefit, or the amount that I am receiving changes or stops, or I receive a lump-sum settlement.
- I am imprisoned for conviction of a felony.

The above events may affect my eligibility to disability benefits as provided in the Social Security Act, as amended.

I know that anyone who makes or causes to be made a false statement or representation of material fact in an application or for use in determining a right to payment under the Social Security Act commits a crime punishable under Federal law by fine, imprisonment or both. I affirm that all information I have given in this document is true.

SIGNATURE OF APPLICANT	Date (Month, day, year)
Signature (First name, middle initial, last name) (Write in ink)	

SIGN HERE ▶

Telephone Number(s) at which you may be contacted during the day. (Include the area code)

FOR OFFICIAL USE ONLY	Direct Deposit Payment Address *(Financial Institution)*		
	Routing Transit Number	C/S	Depositor Account Number

☐ No Account

☐ Direct Deposit Refused

Applicant's Mailing Address *(Number and street, Apt. No., P.O. Box, or Rural Route) (Enter Residence Address in "Remarks," if different.)*

City and State	ZIP Code	County *(if any)* in which you now live

Witnesses are required ONLY if this application has been signed by mark (X) above. If signed by mark (X), two witnesses to the signing who know the applicant must sign below, giving their full addresses. Also, print the applicant's name in Signature block.

1. Signature of Witness	2. Signature of Witness
Address (Number and street, City, State and ZIP Code)	Address (Number and street, City, State and ZIP Code)

Form SSA-16-F6 (7-89)   Page 4

FOR YOUR INFORMATION

An agency in your State that works with us in administering the Social Security disability program is responsible for making the disability decision on your claim. In some cases, it is necessary for them to get additional information about your condition or to arrange for you to have a medical examination at Government expense.

RECEIPT FOR YOUR CLAIM FOR SOCIAL SECURITY DISABILITY INSURANCE BENEFITS

PERSON TO CONTACT ABOUT YOUR CLAIM	SSA OFFICE	DATE CLAIM RECEIVED

TELEPHONE NUMBER (INCLUDE AREA CODE)

Your application for Social Security disability benefits has been received and will be processed as quickly as possible.

You should hear from use within _____ days after you have given us all the information we requested. Some claims may take longer if additional information is needed.

In the meantime, if you change your address, or if there is some other change that may affect your claim, you - or someone for you - should report the change. The changes to be reported are listed below.

Always give us your claim number when writing or telephoning about your claim.

If you have any questions about your claim, we will be glad to help you.

CLAIMANT	SOCIAL SECURITY CLAIM NUMBER

CHANGES TO BE REPORTED AND HOW TO REPORT
FAILURE TO REPORT MAY RESULT IN OVERPAYMENTS THAT MUST BE REPAID

➤ You change your mailing address for checks or residence. To avoid delay in receipt of checks you should ALSO file a regular change of address notice with your post office.

➤ You go outside the U.S.A. for 30 consecutive days or longer.

➤ Any beneficiary dies or becomes unable to handle benefits.

➤ Custody Change—Report if a person for whom you are filing or who is in your care dies, leaves your care or custody, or changes address.

➤ You are confined to jail, prison, penal institution, or correctional facility for conviction of a felony.

➤ You become entitled to a pension or annuity based on your employment after 1956 not covered by Social Security, or if such pension or annuity stops.

➤ Change of Marital Status—Marriage, divorce, annulment of marriage.

➤ You return to work (as an employee or self-employed) regardless of amount of earnings.

➤ Your condition improves.

➤ If you apply for or begin to receive workers' compensation (including black lung benefits) or another public disability benefit, or the amount of your present workers' compensation or public disability benefit changes or stops, or you receive a lump-sum settlement.

HOW TO REPORT
You can make your reports by telephone, mail, or in person, whichever you prefer.

If you are awarded benefits, and one or more of the above changes occur, the change(s) should be reported by calling:

(Telephone Number—Include Area Code)

☆U S GPO 1990-261-237/00059

TO BE COMPLETED BY SSA
NUMBER HOLDER

SOCIAL SECURITY NUMBER

EMPLOYEE/CLAIMANT/BENEFICIARY (If other than Number Holder)

AUTHORIZATION FOR SOURCE TO RELEASE
INFORMATION TO THE SOCIAL SECURITY ADMINISTRATION (SSA)

INFORMATION ABOUT SOURCE— PLEASE PRINT, TYPE, OR WRITE CLEARLY

NAME AND ADDRESS OF SOURCE (Include Zip Code)	RELATIONSHIP TO CLAIMANT/BENEFICIARY

INFORMATION ABOUT CLAIMANT/BENEFICIARY – PLEASE PRINT, TYPE, OR WRITE CLEARLY

NAME AND ADDRESS (If known) AT TIME CLAIMANT/BENEFICIARY HAD CONTACT WITH SOURCE (Include Zip Code)	DATE OF BIRTH	CLAIMANT/BENEFICIARY I.D. NUMBER (If known and different than SSN) (Clinic/Patient No.)

APPROXIMATE DATES OF CLAIMANT/BENEFICIARY CONTACT WITH SOURCE (e.g., dates of hospital admission, treatment, discharge, etc.)

TO BE COMPLETED BY CLAIMANT/BENEFICIARY OR PERSON AUTHORIZED TO ACT IN HIS/HER BEHALF

GENERAL AND SPECIAL AUTHORIZATION TO RELEASE MEDICAL AND OTHER INFORMATION IN ACCORDANCE WITH THE PROVISIONS OF THE SOCIAL SECURITY ACT; THE PUBLIC HEALTH SERVICE ACT, SECTIONS 523 AND 527; AND TITLE 38 U.S.C. VETERANS BENEFITS, SECTION 4132.

I hereby authorize the above-named source to release or disclose to the Social Security Administration or State agency the following information for the period(s) identified above:

1) All medical records or other information regarding my treatment, hospitalization, and/or outpatient care for my impairment(s), including psychological or psychiatric impairment(s), drug abuse, alcoholism, sickle cell anemia, acquired immunodeficiency syndrome (AIDS), or tests for or infection with human immunodeficiency virus (HIV);

2) Information about how my impairment(s) affects my ability to complete tasks and activities of daily living;

3) Information about how my impairment(s) affected my ability to work.

I understand that this authorization, except for action already taken, may be voided by me at anytime. If I do not void this authorization, it will automatically end when a final decision is made on my claim. If I am already receiving benefits, the authorization will end when a final decision is made as to whether I can continue to receive benefits.

READ IMPORTANT INFORMATION ON REVERSE BEFORE SIGNING FORM BELOW.

SIGNATURE OF CLAIMANT/BENEFICIARY OR PERSON AUTHORIZED TO ACT IN HIS/HER BEHALF	RELATIONSHIP TO CLAIMANT/ BENEFICIARY	DATE
STREET ADDRESS	TELEPHONE NUMBER (Area Code)	
CITY	STATE	ZIP CODE

The signature and address of a person who either knows the person signing this form or is satisfied as to that person's identity is requested below. This is not required by the Social Security Administration, but without it the source may not honor this authorization.

SIGNATURE OF WITNESS	STREET ADDRESS	
CITY	STATE	ZIP CODE

Form SSA-827 (1-91) Use Prior Editions   **(OVER)**

Explanation of Form SSA-827, Authorization For Source to Release Information to the Social Security Administration (SSA)

We are requesting that you authorize the release of information about your impairment to us. Sources usually require this authorization before releasing information to us. Also, the law requires this authorization for release of information about certain conditions.

You can provide this authorization by signing a Form SSA-827, Authorization For Source to Release Information to the Social Security Administration (SSA), for each source identified during your disability interview or during the processing of your claim. We must inform you that because of various Federal disclosure laws, SSA cannot give an absolute pledge of confidentiality regarding information submitted in connection with your claim.

PRIVACY ACT NOTICE

The Social Security Administration is authorized to collect the information on this form under sections 205(a), 223(d) and 1631(e)(1) of the Social Security Act. The information on this form is needed by Social Security to make a decision on your claim. While giving us the information on this form is voluntary, failure to provide all or part of the requested information could prevent an accurate or timely decision on your claim and could result in the loss of benefits. Although the information you furnish on this form is almost never used for any purpose other than making a determination on your disability claim, such information may be disclosed by the Social Security Administration as follows:

(1) To enable a third party or agency to assist Social Security in establishing rights to Social Security benefits and/or coverage;

(2) to comply with Federal laws requiring the release of information from Social Security records (e.g., the General Accounting Office and the Department of Veterans Affairs); and

(3) to facilitate statistical research and audit activities necessary to assure the integrity and improvement of the Social Security programs (e.g., to the Bureau of the Census and private concerns under contract to Social Security).

We may also use the information you give us when we match records by computer. Matching programs compare our records with those of other Federal, State, or local government agencies. Many agencies may use matching programs to find or prove that a person qualifies for benefits paid by the Federal government. The law allows us to do this even if you do not agree to it.

These and other reasons why information about you may be used or given out are explained in the **Federal Register**. If you want to learn more about this, contact any Social Security office.

TIME IT TAKES TO COMPLETE THIS FORM

We estimate that it will take you about 8 minutes to complete this form. This includes the time it will take you to read the instructions, gather the necessary facts and fill out the form. If you have comments or suggestions on this estimate, or on any other aspect of this form, write to the Social Security Administration, ATTN: Reports Clearance Officer, 1-A-21 Operations Bldg., Baltimore, MD 21235, and to the Office of Management and Budget, Paperwork Reduction Project, Washington, DC. 20503. **Do not send completed forms or information concerning your claim to these offices.**

'U.S. Government Printing Office: 1991 — 281-908/40007

Social Security
Notice of Disapproved Claim

From: Department of Health and Human Services
      Social Security Administration

Date:

Claim Number:

We have determined that you are not entitled to disability insurance benefits. The reason you are not entitled is that you do not meet the earnings requirement of the law at the time you state you became disabled or at any later date.

It is important for you to know that we have not made any determination as to whether or not you are disabled within the meaning of the law. Since you do not meet the earnings requirement, it has not been necessary to decide whether you meet the disability requirement. An explanation of the earnings requirement is given on the back of this notice.

If you think we are wrong, you can ask that the determination be looked at by a different person. This is called a reconsideration. IF YOU WANT A RECONSIDERATION, YOU MUST ASK FOR IT WITHIN 60 DAYS FROM THE DATE YOU RECEIVE THIS NOTICE. IF YOU WAIT MORE THAN 60 DAYS, YOU MUST GIVE US A GOOD REASON FOR THE DELAY. Your request must be made in writing through any Social Security office. Be sure to tell us your name, Social Security number and why you think we are wrong. If you cannot write to us, call a Social Security office or come in and someone will help you. You can give us more facts to add to your file. However, if you do not have the evidence yet, you should not wait for it before asking for a reconsideration. You may send the evidence in later. We will then decide your case again. You will not meet with the person who will decide your case. Please read the enclosed leaflet for a full explanation of your right to appeal.

You have the right to file a new application at any time, but filing a new application is not the same as appealing this decision. You might lose benefits if you file a new application instead of filing an appeal. Therefore, if you think this decision is wrong, you should ask for an appeal within 60 days.

If you have questions about your claim, you may get in touch with any Social Security office. Most questions can be handled by telephone or mail. If you visit an office, however, please take this letter with you.

Enclosures:
SSA Publication No. 05-10058
SSA Publication No. 05-10072

Important: See other side for additional information. ➤

Form SSA-L807.5-U2 (12/89)
DESTROY PRIOR EDITIONS

Important Information

A person may qualify for Social Security disability insurance benefits only if the person meets both the earnings requirement and the disability requirement of the law. These two requirements are explained below.

The Earnings Requirement

➤ A person whose disability began before age 24 meets the earnings requirement if Social Security credits have been earned for 6 calendar quarters (1 ½ years) of work during the 12-quarter (3-year) period ending with a quarter before age 24 in which the disability exists.

➤ A person whose disability began between the ages 24 and 31 meets the earnings requirement if Social Security credits have been earned for work in at least one-half of the calendar quarters in the period beginning with the calendar quarter after age 21 and ending with a quarter before age 31 in which the disability exists.

➤ A person whose disability began at age 31 or later needs to meet the two provisions of the earnings requirement shown below:

(1) Credit for 20 calendar quarters (5 years) of work during a 40-quarter period (10 years) ending in or after a quarter in which disability exists.

(2) Credit for one calendar quarter of work for each year after 1950 (or after reaching age 21, if that is later) up to the year the disability began. In this second instance, the credits do not have to have been earned during the past 10 years.

➤ A person who had a period of disability which began before age 31 and later ended, and who became disabled again before, or after age 31, can meet the earnings requirement if he/she had one quarter of coverage for every two calendar quarters after age 21 and through the quarter in which the later period of disability began, excluding the prior period of disability.

A person who does not have credit for the amount of work shown above is not eligible for disability insurance benefits under the Social Security Act.

The Disability Requirement

To be considered disabled, a person must be unable to do any substantial gainful work due to a medical condition which has lasted or is expected to last for at least 12 months in a row. The condition must be severe enough to keep a person from working not only in his or her usual job, but in any other substantial gainful work. We look at the person's age, education, training and work experience when we decide whether he or she can work.

Other Disability Programs

Definitions of disability are not the same in all government and private disability programs. Government agencies must follow the laws that apply to their own disability programs. A finding by a private organization or other government agency that a person is disabled does not necessarily mean that the person meets the disability requirements of the Social Security Act.

Family Benefits

No benefits may be paid to a wife, husband, or child unless the wage earner or self-employed person is entitled to Social Security disability insurance benefits.

REQUEST FOR RECONSIDERATION

(Do not wirte in this space)

The information on this form is authorized by regulation (20 CFR 404.907 -- 404.921 and 416.1407 -- 416.1421). While your responses to these questions is voluntary, the Social Security Administration cannot reconsider the decision on this claim unless the information is furnished.

NAME OF CLAIMANT	NAME OF WAGE EARNER OR SELF-EMPLOYED PERSON *(If different from claimant.)*
SOCIAL SECURITY CLAIM NUMBER	SUPPLEMENTAL SECURITY INCOME (SSI) CLAIM NUMBER
SPOUSE'S NAME *(Complete ONLY in SSI cases)*	SPOUSE'S SOCIAL SECURITY NUMBER *(Complete ONLY in SSI cases)*

CLAIM FOR *(Specify type, e.g., retirement, disability, hospital insurance, SSI, etc.)*

I do not agree with the determination made on the above claim and request reconsideration. My reasons are:

SUPPLEMENTAL SECURITY INCOME RECONSIDERATION ONLY *(See reverse of claimant's copy)*

"I want to appeal your decision about my claim for supplemental security income, SSI. I've read the back of this form about the three ways to appeal. I've checked the box below."

☐ Case Review   ☐ Informal Conference   ☐ Formal Conference

EITHER THE CLAIMANT OR REPRESENTATIVE SHOULD SIGN -- ENTER ADDRESSES FOR BOTH

SIGNATURE OR NAME OF CLAIMANT'S REPRESENTATIVE ☐ NON-ATTORNEY ☐ ATTORNEY	CLAIMANT SIGNATURE
STREET ADDRESS	STREET ADDRESS
CITY STATE ZIP CODE	CITY STATE ZIP CODE
TELEPHONE NUMBER *(Include area code)* (_ _ _) DATE	TELEPHONE NUMBER *(Include area code)* (_ _ _) DATE

TO BE COMPLETED BY SOCIAL SECURITY ADMINISTRATION

See reverse of claim folder copy for list of initial determinations

1. HAS INITIAL DETERMINATION BEEN MADE? ☐ YES ☐ NO	2. CLAIMANT INSISTS ON FILING ☐ YES ☐ NO

3. IS THIS REQUEST FILED TIMELY? ☐ YES ☐ NO
(If "NO", attach claimant's explanation for delay and attach only pertinent letter, material, or information in social security office.)

RETIREMENT AND SURVIVORS RECONSIDERATIONS ONLY (CHECK ONE) REFER TO (GN 03102.125) | SOCIAL SECURITY OFFICE ADDRESS

☐ NO FURTHER DEVELOPMENT REQUIRED   (GN 03102.125)

☐ REQUIRED DEVELOPMENT ATTACHED

☐ REQUIRED DEVELOPMENT PENDING, WILL FORWARD OR ADVISE STATUS WITHIN 30 DAYS

ROUTING INSTRUCTIONS (CHECK ONE)

☐ DISABILITY DETERMINATION SERVICES *(ROUTE WITH DISABILITY FOLDER)*   ☐ ODO, BALTIMORE   ☐ PROGRAM SERVICE CENTER

☐ INTPSC, BALTIMORE   ☐ DISTRICT OFFICE RECONSIDERATION   ☐ OCRO BALTIMORE

NOTE: TAKE OR MAIL COMPLETED COPIES TO YOUR SOCIAL SECURITY OFFICE

FORM **SSA-561-U2** (9-85)   CLAIMS FOLDER

ADMINISTRATIVE ACTIONS THAT ARE INITIAL DETERMINATIONS
(See GN 03101.190, GN 03101.200, and GN 03110.210)

NOTE: These lists cover the vast majority of administrative actions that are initial determinations. However, they are not all inclusive.

Title II

1. Entitlement or continuing entitlement to benefits;
2. Reentitlement to benefits;
3. The amount of benefit;
4. A recomputation of benefit;
5. A reduction in disability benefits because benefits under a worker's compensation law was also received;
6. A deduction from benefits on account of work;
7. A deduction from disability benefits because of claimant's refusal to accept rehabilitation services;
8. Termination of benefits;
9. Penalty deductions imposed because of failure to report certain events;
10. Any overpayment or underpayment of benefits;
11. Whether an overpayment of benefits must be repaid;
12. How an underpayment of benefits due a deceased person will be paid;
13. The establishment or termination of a period of disability;
14. A revision of an earnings record;
15. Whether the payment of benefits will be made, on the claimant's behalf to a representative payee, unless the claimant is under age 18 or legally imcompetent;
16. Who will act as the payee if we determine that representative payment will be made;
17. An offset of benefits because the claimant previously received Supplemental Security Income payments for the same period;
18. Whether completion of or continuation for a specified period of time in an appropriate vocational rehabilitation program will significantly increase the likelihood that the claimant will not have to return to the disability benefit rolls and thus, whether the claimant's benefits may be continued even though the claimant is not disabled; and

19. Nonpayment of benefits because of claimant's confinement in a jail, prison, or other penal institution or correctional facility for conviction of a felony.

Title XVI

1. Eligibility for, or the amount of, Supplement Security Income benefits;
2. Suspension, reduction, or termination of Supplemental Security Income benefits;
3. Whether an overpayment of benefits must be repaid;
4. Whether payments will be made, on claimant's behalf to a representative payee, unless the claimant is under age 18, legally incompetent, or determined to be a drug addict or alcoholic;
5. Who will act as payee if we determine that representative payment will be made;
6. Imposing penalties for failing to report improtant information;
7. Drug addiction or alcoholism;
8. Whether claimant is eligible for special SSI cash benefits;
9. Whether claimant is eligible for special SSI eligibility status;
10. Claimant's disability; and
11. Whether completion of or continuation for a specified period of time in an appropriate vocational rehabilitation program will significantly increase the likelihood that claimant will not have to return to the disability benefit rolls and thus, whether claimant's benefits may be continued even though he or she is not disabled.

NOTE: Every redetermination which gives an individual the right of further review constitutes an initial determination.

Title XVIII

1. Entitlement to hospital insurance benefits and to enrollment for supplementary medical insurance benefits;
2. Disallowance (including denial of application for HIB and denial of application for enrollment for SMIB);
3. Termination of benefits (including termination of entitlement to HI and SMI).

DEPARTMENT OF HEALTH AND HUMAN SERVICES
Social Security Administration

Form Approved
OMB No. 0960-0144

For SSA Use Only - Do NOT Complete This Item.	
Name of Wage Earner	Social Security Number
Name of Claimant	Social Security Number

Type of Claim:

Title II — ☐ Freeze ☐ DIB ☐ DWB ☐ CDB Title XVI — ☐ Disability ☐ Blind ☐ Child

RECONSIDERATION DISABILITY REPORT

PLEASE PRINT, TYPE, OR WRITE CLEARLY AND ANSWER ALL ITEMS TO THE BEST OF YOUR ABILITY. If you are filing on behalf of someone else, answer all questions. COMPLETE ANSWERS WILL AID IN PROCESSING THE CLAIM.

Privacy Act/Paperwork Act Notice: Your response to this request is voluntary, however failure to provide all or any part of the requested information may affect the final decision on your claim. The information you provide will be used to augment the medical evidence in your case. The information requested on this form is authorized by section 404.1512 and 416.912 of the Social Security regulations. Information you furnish on this form may be disclosed by the Social Security Administration to another person or governmental agency only with respect to social security programs and to comply with Federal laws requiring the exchange of information between the Social Security Administration and another agency.

Date Claim Filed [   ]

PART I — INFORMATION ABOUT YOUR CONDITION

1. Has there been any change (for better or worse) in your illness or injury since you filed your claim? .... ☐ Yes ☐ No
If "Yes," describe any changes in your symptoms.

2. Describe any physical or mental limitations you have as a result of your condition, since you filed your claim.

3. Have any restrictions been placed on you by a physician since you filed your claim? .... ☐ Yes ☐ No
If "Yes," give name, address, and telephone number of the physician and show what kinds of restrictions have been imposed.

4. Do you have any additional illness or injury that you feel we should know about? .... ☐ Yes ☐ No
If "Yes," describe the kind of illness or injury and the date that it occurred.

Form SSA-3441-F6 (5-86) Prior editions may be used   1

PART II — INFORMATION ABOUT YOUR MEDICAL RECORDS

5. Have you seen any physician since you filed your claim? .... ☐ Yes   ☐ No
   If "Yes," provide the following about the physician you last visited:

NAME	ADDRESS (Include ZIP Code)
AREA CODE AND TELEPHONE NUMBER	
HOW OFTEN DO YOU SEE THIS PHYSICIAN	DATES YOU SAW THIS PHYSICIAN
REASONS FOR VISITS	

TYPE OF TREATMENT RECEIVED (Include drugs, surgery, tests)

6. Have you seen any other physician since you filed your claim? .... ☐ Yes   ☐ No
   If "Yes," show the following:

NAME	ADDRESS (Include ZIP Code)
AREA CODE AND TELEPHONE NUMBER	
HOW OFTEN DO YOU SEE THIS PHYSICIAN?	DATES YOU SAW THIS PHYSICIAN
REASONS FOR VISITS	

TYPE OF TREATMENT RECEIVED (Include drugs, surgery, tests)

If you have seen other physicians since you filed your claim, list their names, addresses, dates and reasons for visits in Part V.

7. Have you been hospitalized, or treated at a clinic or confined in a nursing home or
   extended care facility for your illness or injury since you filed your claim? .... ☐ Yes   ☐ No
   If "Yes," show the following:

NAME OF FACILITY	ADDRESS OF AGENCY (Include ZIP Code)
PATIENT OR CLINIC NUMBER	

WERE YOU AN INPATIENT? (Stayed at least overnight)	DATES OF ADMISSIONS AND DISCHARGES
☐ Yes ☐ No IF "YES," SHOW ⟶	
WERE YOU AN OUTPATIENT?	DATES OF VISITS
☐ Yes ☐ No IF "YES" SHOW ⟶	

REASON FOR HOSPITALIZATION, CLINIC VISITS, OR CONFINEMENT

TYPE OF TREATMENT RECEIVED (Include drugs, surgery, tests)

If you have been in other hospitals, clinics, nursing homes, or extended care facilities for your illness or injury, list the names, addresses, patient or clinic numbers, dates and reasons for hospitalization, clinic visits, or confinement in Part V.

8. Have you been seen by other agencies for your injury or illness? .... ☐ Yes   ☐ No
   (VA, Workmen's Compensation, Vocational Rehabilitation, Welfare, Special Schools, Unions, etc.)
   If "Yes," show the following:

NAME OF AGENCY	ADDRESS OF AGENCY (Including ZIP Code)
YOUR CLAIM NUMBER	
DATES OF VISITS	NAME OF COUNSELOR, SOCIAL WORKER, ETC.

TYPE OF TREATMENT OR EXAMINATION RECEIVED (Include drugs, surgery, tests)

If more space is needed, list the other agencies, their addresses, your claim numbers, dates, and treatment received in Part V.

Form SSA-3441-F6 (5-86)   2

PART III — INFORMATION ABOUT WORK

9. Have you worked since you filed your claim? .... ☐ Yes   ☐ No

   If "Yes," you will be asked to give details on a separate form.

PART IV — INFORMATION ABOUT YOUR ACTIVITIES

10. How does your illness or injury affect your ability to care for your personal needs?

11. What changes have occurred in your daily activities since you filed your claim?
    (If none, show, "None")

PART V — REMARKS AND AUTHORIZATIONS

12.(a) READ CAREFULLY: I authorize the Social Security Administration to release information from my records, as necessary to process my claim, as follows:

   Copies of my medical records may be furnished to a physician or a medical institution for background information if it is necessary for me to have a medical examination by that physician or medical institution. The results of any such examination may be given to my personal physician.

   Information from my records may also be furnished, if necessary, to any company providing clerical and administrative services for the purposes of transcribing, typing, copying or otherwise clerically servicing such information. The State Vocational Rehabilitation Agency may also have access to information in my records to determine my eligibility for rehabilitative services.

   I understand and concur with the statement and authorizations given above, except as follows (If there are no exceptions, write "None" in the space below. If you do not concur with any part of the above statement, state your objections clearly):

12. (b)	Telephone number where you can be reached:	Best time to reach you:

Form SSA-3441-F6 (5-86)   3

12(b) Use this section to continue information required by prior sections. Identify the section for which the information is provided.

Note: This section may also be used for any special or additional information which you wish to be recorded

_____

_____

_____

_____

_____

_____

_____

_____

_____

_____

_____

_____

_____

_____

_____

_____

_____

_____

_____

_____

Knowing that anyone making a false statement or representation of a material fact for use in determining a right to payment under the Social Security Act commits a crime punishable under Federal Law, I certify that the above statements are true.

NAME (SIGNATURE OF CLAIMANT OR PERSON FILING ON THE CLAIMANT'S BEHALF)

SIGN HERE ▶ | DATE

Name of Wage Earner	Social Security Number
Name of Claimant	Social Security Number

13. Check each item to indicate whether or not any difficulty was observed:
    (Explain all items checked "Yes," in Item 14 below)

Reading:	☐ Yes	☐ No	Using Hands:	☐ Yes	☐ No
Writing:	☐ Yes	☐ No	Breathing:	☐ Yes	☐ No
Answering:	☐ Yes	☐ No	Seeing:	☐ Yes	☐ No
Hearing:	☐ Yes	☐ No	Walking:	☐ Yes	☐ No
Speaking:	☐ Yes	☐ No	Sitting	☐ Yes	☐ No
Understanding:	☐ Yes	☐ No	Assistive Devices:	☐ Yes	☐ No

Other *(Specify)*: _____

14. If any of the above items were checked "Yes," describe the observed difficulty:

15. Describe fully: General appearance, behavior, any unusual observed difficulties not noted elsewhere, any unusual circumstances surrounding the interviews.

Form **SSA-3441-F6** (5-86)   5

16. Claimant requires assistance .... ☐ Yes   ☐ No
If "Yes," show name, address, phone number, and relationship of interested person.
Also show why claimant requires assistance (foreign-speaking, unable to ambulate, etc.)

17. Capability development appears needed .... ☐ Yes   ☐ No
If "Yes," indicate whether DO will undertake development because it is also developing
medical evidence from a special arrangement source. (Show name and address of source.)

18. Is development of work activity necessary? .... ☐ Yes   ☐ No

If "Yes," is an SSA-821 or SSA-820-F4 ☐ Pending   ☐ In File

19. SSA-3441 Taken By:
☐ Personal Interview
  ☐ DO/BO ☐ Home ☐ Other _____
☐ Telephone
☐ Mail

Signature of Interviewer or Reviewer	Title	DO, BO, or TSC	Date

Form SSA-3441-F6 (5-86)   6   ☆ U.S. Government Printing Office: 1986—491-371/20118

31515.240 SSA-L928-U2

A. Front

Social Security
Notice of Reconsideration

From: Department of Health and Human Services
          Social Security Administration

Date:

Claim Number:

Claim for
☐ Disability Insurance Benefits
☐ Disabled Widow, Widower Benefits
☐ Childhood Disability Benefits
☐ Medicare Coverage Only

Upon receipt of your request for reconsideration we had your claim independently reviewed by a physician and disability examiner in the State agency which works with us in making disability determinations. The evidence in your case has been thoroughly evaluated; this includes the medical evidence and the additional information received since the original decision. We find that the previous determination denying your claim was proper under the law. Attached to this notice is an explanation of the decision we made on your claim and how we arrived at it. The reverse of this notice identifies the legal requirements for your type of claim.

The determination on your claim was made by an agency of the State. It was not made by your own doctor or by other people or agencies writing reports about you. However, any evidence they gave us was used in making this determination. Doctors and other people in the State agency who are trained in disability evaluation reviewed the evidence and made the determination based on Social Security law and regulations.

If you believe that the reconsideration determination is not correct, you may request a hearing before an administrative law judge of the Office of Hearings and Appeals. If you want a hearing, you must request it not later than 60 days from the date you receive this notice. You may make your request through any Social Security office. Read the enclosed leaflet for a full explanation of your right to appeal.

If you do not request a hearing of your case within the prescribed time period, you still have the right to file another application at any time.

This decision refers only to your claim for benefits under the Social Security Disability Insurance Program. If you applied for other benefits, you will receive a separate notice when a decision is made on that claim(s).

If you have questions about your claim, you should get in touch with any Social Security office. Most questions can be handled by telephone or mail. If you visit an office, however, please take this letter with you.

Enclosure:
SSA Pub. No. 70-10282

Important: See other side for additional information. ▶

Form SSA-L928-U2 (3-85)
Prior editions may be used until supply is exhausted

B. Reverse

Summarized below are legal requirements for the various types of disability claims:

Disability Insurance Claim
To be considered disabled, a person must be unable to do any substantial gainful work due to a medical condition which has lasted or is expected to last for a least 12 months in a row. The condition must be severe enough to keep a person from working not only in his or her usual job, but in any other substantial gainful work. We look at the person's age, education, training and work experience when we decide whether he or she can work.

Disabled Widow (Widower) Claim
A widow, widower, or surviving divorced wife (age 50-60) must meet the disability requirement of the law within a specified 7-year period. A person may be considered disabled only if he or she has a physical or mental impairment that is so severe as to ordinarily prevent a person from working. The disability must have lasted or be expected to last for a continuous period of at least 12 months.

Childhood Disability Benefits
Childhood disability benefits may be paid to a person age 18 or older in the person has a disability which began before age 22 or within 84 months of the end of an earlier period of childhood disability. The condition, whether physical or mental, must be severe enough to keep the person from doing any substantial gainful work. We look at the person's age, education and previous training when we decide whether he or she can work. In addition, the condition must have lasted or be expected to last for a least 12 months in a row.

259

Form Approved
OMB No. 0960-0318

CLAIMANT'S STATEMENT WHEN REQUEST FOR HEARING IS FILED AND THE ISSUE IS DISABILITY

Print, type or write clearly and answer all questions to the best of your ability. Complete answers will aid in processing the claim. IF ADDITIONAL SPACE IS NEEDED, ATTACH A SEPARATE STATEMENT TO THIS FORM.

CLAIMANT'S NAME	SOCIAL SECURITY NUMBER
WAGE EARNER (LEAVE BLANK IF NAME IS THE SAME AS THE CLAIMANT'S)	SOCIAL SECURITY NUMBER

PRIVACEY ACT AND PAPERWORK ACT NOTICE: The Social Security Act (sections 205(a), 702, 1631(e)(1)(A) and (B), and 1869(b)(1) and (c), as appropriate authorizes the collection of information on this form. We will use the information on your recent activities, condition, medical treatment, and medications to help us decide if we need to obtain more information. You do not have to give it, but if you do not you may not receive benefits under the Social Security Act. We may give out the information on this form without your written consent if we need to get more information to decide if you are eligible for benefits or if a Federal law requires us to do so. Specifically, we may provide information to another Federal, State, or local government agency which is deciding your eligibility for a government benefit or program; to the President or a Congressman inquiring on your behalf; to an independent party who needs statistical information for a research paper or audit report on a Social Security program; or to the Department of Justice to represent the Federal Government in a court suit related to a program administered by the Social Security Administration.

We may also use the information you give us when we match records by computer. Matching programs compare our records with those of other Federal, State, or local government agencies. Many agencies may use matching programs to find or prove that a person qualifies for benefits paid by the Federal government. The law allows us to do this even if you do not agree to it.

These and other reasons why information about you may be used or given out are explained in the Federal Register. If you want to learn more about this, contact any Social Security Office.

TIME IT TAKES TO COMPLETE THIS FORM

We estimate that it will take you about 15 minutes to complete this form. This includes the time it will take to read the instructions, gather the necessary facts and fill out the form. If you have comments or suggestions on how long it takes to complete this form or on any other aspect of this form, write to the Social Security Administration, ATTN: Reports Clearance Officer, 1-A-21 Operations Bldg., Baltimore, MD 21235, and to the Office of Management and Budget, Paperwork Reduction Project (0960-0318), Washington, D.C. 20503. Do not send completed forms or information concerning your claim to these offices.

1. Have you worked since _____, the date your request for reconsideration was filed? (If yes, describe the nature and exent of work.) ⟶ ☐ Yes ☐ No

2. Has there been any change in your condition since the above date? (If yes, describe the change.) ⟶ ☐ Yes ☐ No

3. Have your daily activities and/or social functioning changed since the above date? (If yes, describe the changes.) ⟶ ☐ Yes ☐ No

4. Have you been treated or examined by a doctor (other than as a patient in a hospital) since the above date? (If yes, complete the following.) ⟶ ☐ Yes ☐ No

NAME AND ADDRESS OF DOCTOR(S)	DATE OF EXAM	MEDICAL PROBLEM

Form HA-4486 (9/90) (OVER)

5. Have you been a patient in a hospital since the above date? (If yes, complete the following.) ⟶   ☐ Yes   ☐ No

NAME AND ADDRESS OF HOSPITAL(S)	DATE OF HOSPITALIZATION	MEDICAL PROBLEM

6. Have you received medical or vocational services from a community agency since the above date? ⟶   ☐ Yes   ☐ No

7. Are you now taking any prescription drugs or medications? (If yes, list them below.) ⟶   ☐ Yes   ☐ No

NAME OF MEDICATION(S)	DOSAGE BEING TAKEN	NAME OF PHYSICIAN(S)

8. Are you now taking any nonprescription drugs or medications? (If yes, list them below.)   ☐ Yes   ☐ No

NAME OF MEDICATION(S)	DOSAGE BEING TAKEN

Knowing that anyone making a false statement or representation of a material fact for use in determining a right to payment under the Social Security Act commits a crime punishable under Federal Law, I certify that the above statements are true.

SIGNATURE OF CLAIMANT OR PERSON FILING ON THE CLAIMANT'S BEHALF	DATE SIGNED
SIGN HERE ▶	

DEPARTMENT OF HEALTH AND HUMAN SERVICES
SOCIAL SECURITY ADMINISTRATION
OFFICE OF HEARINGS AND APPEALS

261 Form Approved
OMB No. 0960-0269

REQUEST FOR HEARING BY ADMINISTRATIVE LAW JUDGE
[Take or mail original and all copies to your local Social Security Office]

PRIVACY ACT NOTICE
ON REVERSE SIDE OF FORM.

1. CLAIMANT	2. WAGE EARNER, IF DIFFERENT	3. SOC SEC CLAIM NUMBER	4 SPOUSE's CLAIM NUMBER

5. I REQUEST A HEARING BEFORE AN ADMINISTRATIVE LAW JUDGE. I disagree with the determination made on my claim because:

You have a right to be represented at the hearing. If you are not represented but would like to be, your Social Security Office will give you a list of legal referral and service organizations. (If you are represented, complete form SSA-1696.)

An Administrative Law Judge of the Office of Hearings and Appeals will be appointed to conduct the hearing or other proceedings in your case. You will receive notice of the time and place of a hearing at least 20 days before the day set for a hearing.

6. Check one of these blocks.

☐ I have no additional evidence to submit.

☐ I have additional evidence to submit.
(Please submit it to the Social
Security Office within 10 days.)

7. Check one of the blocks:

☐ I wish to appear at a hearing.

☐ I do not wish to appear and I request that a decision be made based on the evidence in my case.
(Complete Waiver Form HA-4608)

[You should complete No. 8 and your representative (if any) should complete No. 9. If you are represented and your representative is not available to complete this form, you should also print his or her name, address, etc. in No. 9.]

8.	9.
(CLAIMANT'S SIGNATURE)	(REPRESENTATIVE'S SIGNATURE/NAME)
ADDRESS	(ADDRESS) ☐ ATTORNEY; ☐ NON ATTORNEY
CITY STATE ZIP CODE	CITY STATE ZIP CODE
DATE AREA CODE AND TELEPHONE NUMBER	DATE AREA CODE AND TELEPHONE NUMBER

TO BE COMPLETED BY SOCIAL SECURITY ADMINISTRATION–ACKNOWLEDGMENT OF REQUEST FOR HEARING

10.
Request for Hearing RECEIVED for the Social Security Administration on _____ by: _____

(TITLE)	ADDRESS	Servicing FO Code	PC Code

11.
☐ Request timely field.

☐ Request not timely filed-Attach (1) claimant's explanation for delay, (2) any pertinent letter, material, or information in the Social/Security Office.

12. Claimant not represented –
☐ list of legal referral and service organizations provided

13. Interpreter needed–
☐ enter language (including sign language): _____

14.
Check one: ☐ Initial Entitlement Case
☐ Disability Cessation Case
☐ Other Postentitlement Case

15.
Check claim type(s):
☐ RSI only ....(RSI)
☐ Disability–worker or child only ....(DIWC)
☐ Disability–Widow(er) only ....(DIWW)
☐ SSI Aged only ....(SSIA)
☐ SSI Blind only ....(SSIB)
☐ SSI Disability only ....(SSID)
☐ SSI Aged/Title II ....(SSAC)
☐ SSI Blind/Title II ....(SSBC)
☐ SSI Disability/Title II ....(SSDC)
☐ HI Entitlement ....(HIE)
☐ Other–Specify: (_____)

16.
HO COPY SENT TO: _____ HO on _____
☐ CF Attached: ☐ Title II; ☐ Title XVI; or
☐ Title II CF held in FO to establish CAPS ORBIT; or
☐ CF requested: ☐ Title II; ☐ Title XVI
(Copy of teletype or phone report attached).

17.
CF COPY SENT TO: _____ HO on _____
☐ CF attached: ☐ Title II; ☐ Title XVI
☐ Other attached _____

FORM HA-501-U5 (2-87)
Destroy old stock

CLAIMS FOLDER

Form HA-501-U5 (2-87)

Form Approved
OMB No. 0960-0280

ACKNOWLEDGMENT OF NOTICE OF HEARING
(Complete this card and return it at once in the envelope provided. No postage is necessary.)

CLAIMANT	SOCIAL SECURITY NUMBER

WAGE EARNER	HEARING OFFICE

(Check only one)

☐ **I will be present** at the time and place shown on the Notice of Hearing. If an emergency arises after I mail this form and I cannot be present, I will immediately notify you at the telephone number shown on the Notice of Hearing.

☐ **I cannot be present** at the time or place shown on the Notice of Hearing. I request that you reschedule my hearing because: _____

_____

(Use the reverse side for additional remarks.)

NOTE: YOUR REQUEST FOR HEARING MAY BE DISMISSED IF YOU DO NOT ATTEND THE HEARING AND CANNOT GIVE A GOOD REASON FOR NOT ATTENDING. THE TIME OR PLACE OF THE HEARING WILL BE CHANGED IF YOU HAVE A GOOD REASON FOR YOUR REQUEST.

SIGNATURE	DATE	AREA CODE AND TELEPHONE NO.

☐ I have recently moved. My new address is on the reverse side.

Form HA-504 (12/86) Issue 6/86 Edition Until Supply Is Exhausted

PAPERWORK/PRIVACY ACT NOTICE: The collection of information on this form is authorized by sections 205(a), 702, 163¹:(e)(1)(A) and (B), and 1869(b)(1) and (c) of the Social Security Act, as appropriate. The information provided is needed to acknowledge notice of a hearing and will be used to further process your claim. Information requested on this form is voluntary, but failure to provide all or any part of the requested information may affect the decision on your claim. Information you furnish on this form may be disclosed by the Social Security Administration to another person or government agency only with respect to Social Security programs and to comply with Federal laws requiring the disclosure of information or the exchange of information between the Social Security Administration and other agencies.

Use this space to give the reasons you cannot attend the scheduled hearing or to provide your current address.

NAME (Claimant) (Print or Type) | SOCIAL SECURITY NUMBER

WAGE EARNER (If different) | SOCIAL SECURITY NUMBER

Section I   APPOINTMENT OF REPRESENTATIVE

I appoint this individual _____

(Name and Address)

to act as my representative in connection with my claim or asserted right under:

☐ Title II
(RSDI)

☐ Title XVI
(SSI)

☐ Title IV FMSHA
(Black Lung)

☐ Title XVIII
(Medicare Coverage)

I authorize this individual to make or give any request or notice; to present or elicit evidence; to obtain information; and to receive any notice in connection with my pending claim or asserted right wholly in my stead.

SIGNATURE (Claimant) | ADDRESS

TELEPHONE NUMBER | DATE

(Area Code)

Section II   ACCEPTANCE OF APPOINTMENT

I, _____ , hereby accept the above appointment. I certify that I have not been suspended or prohibited from practice before the Social Security Administration; that I am not, as a current or former officer or employee of the United States, disqualified from acting as the claimant's representative; and that I will not charge or receive any fee for the representation unless it has been authorized in accordance with the laws and regulations referred to on the reverse side hereof. In the event that I decide not to charge or collect a fee for the representation, I will notify the Social Security Administration. (Completion of Section III satisfies this requirement.)

I am a / an _____

(Attorney, union representative, relative, law student, etc.)

SIGNATURE (Representative) | ADDRESS

TELEPHONE NUMBER | DATE

(Area code)

Section III (Optional)   WAIVER OF FEE

I waive my right to charge and collect a fee under Section 206 of the Social Security Act, and I release my client (the claimant) from any obligations, contractual or otherwise, which may be owed to me for services I have performed in connection with my client's claim or asserted right.

SIGNATURE (Representative) | DATE

WAIVER OF DIRECT PAYMENT

I ONLY waive my right to direct certification of a fee from the withheld past-due benefits of my client (the claimant). I do NOT, however, waive my right to petition for and be authorized to charge and collect a fee directly from my client.

SIGNATURE (Representative) | DATE

Form SSA-1696-U4 (3-88)
Destroy prior editions

(See Important Information on Reverse)

FILE COPY

PRIVACY ACT AND PAPERWORK ACT NOTICE

The Social Security Act (sections 205(a), 702, 1631(e)(1)(A) and (B), and 1869(b)(1) and (c), as appropriate) authorizes the collection of information on this form. We need the information to continue processing your claim. You do not have to give it, but if you do not you may not receive benefits under the Social Security Act. We may give out the information on this form without your written consent if we need to get more information to decide if you are eligible for benefits or if a Federal law requires us to do so. Specifically, we may provide information to another Federal, State, or local government agency which is deciding your eligibility for a government benefit or program; to the President or a Congressman inquiring on your behalf; to an independent party who needs statistical information for a research paper or audit report on a Social Security program; or to the Department of Justice to represent the Federal Government in a court suit related to a program administered by the Social Security Administration. We explain, in the Federal Register, these and other reasons why we may use or give out information about you. If you would like more information, get in touch with any Social Security Office.

FORM **HA-501-U5** (5-88)
Issue old stock

DEPARTMENT OF HEALTH AND HUMAN SERVICES
SOCIAL SECURITY ADMINISTRATION

Form Approved
OMB No. 0960-0104

PETITION TO OBTAIN APPROVAL OF A FEE FOR REPRESENTING A CLAIMANT BEFORE THE SOCIAL SECURITY ADMINISTRATION

IMPORTANT INFORMATION ON REVERSE SIDE

PAPERWORK/PRIVACY ACT NOTICE: Your response to this request is voluntary, but the Social Security Administration may not approve any fee unless it receives the information this form requests. The Administration will use the information to determine a fair value for services you rendered to the claimant named below, as provided in section 206 of the Social Security Act (42 U.S.C. 406).

I request approval to charge a fee of ➤ Fee $ _____ (Show the dollar amount)

for services performed as the representative of _____ ➤ Mr.
Mrs.
Ms. _____

My Services Began: ___/___/___   Type(s) of claim(s) _____
Month Day Year

My Services Ended: ___/___/___

Enter the name and the Social Security number of the person on whose Social Security record the claim is based.

_____ ___/___/___ ___

1.	Itemize on a separate page or pages the services you rendered before the Social Security Administration (SSA). List each meeting, conference, item of correspondence, telephone call, and other activity in which you engaged, such as research, preparation of a brief, attendance at a hearing, travel, etc., related to your services as representative in this case. Attach to this petition the list showing the dates, the descriptions of each service, the actual time spent in each, and the total hours.
2.	Have you and your client entered into a fee agreement for services before SSA? ☐ YES ☐ NO If "yes," please specify the amount on which you agreed, or attach a copy of the agreement to this petition. $ _____ or ☐ See attached
3.	(a) Have you received, or do you expect to receive, any payment toward your fee from any source other than from funds which SSA may be withholding for fee payment? ☐ YES ☐ NO (b) Do you currently hold in a trust or escrow account any amount of money you received toward payment of your fee? ☐ YES ☐ NO If "yes" to either or both of the above, please specify the source(s) and the amount(s). Source: _____ $ _____ Source: _____ $ _____ **Note:** If you receive payment(s) after submitting this petition, but before SSA approves a fee, you have an affirmative duty to notify the SSA office to which you are sending this petition.
4.	Have you received, or do you expect to receive, reimbursement for expenses you incurred? ☐ YES ☐ NO If "yes," please itemize your expenses and the amounts on a separate page.
5.	Did you render any services relating to this matter before any State or Federal court? If "yes," what fee did you or will you charge for services in connection with the court proceeding? ☐ YES ☐ NO $ _____ Please attach a copy of the court order if the court has approved a fee.

I certify that the information above, and on the attachment(s), is true and correct to the best of my knowledge and belief. I also certify that I have furnished a copy of this petition and the attachment(s) to the person(s) for whom I performed the services. I understand that failure to comply with Social Security laws and regulations pertaining to representation may result in suspension or disqualification from practice before SSA, the imposition of criminal penalties, or both.

Signature of Representative _____ Date _____ Address (include Zip Code) _____

Firm with which associated, if any _____ Telephone No. and Area Code _____

[Note: The following is optional. However, SSA can consider your fee petition more promptly if your client knows and already agrees with the amount you are requesting.]

I understand that I do not have to sign this petition or request. It is my right to disagree with the amount of the fee requested or any information given, and to ask more questions about the information given in this request (as explained on the reverse side of this form). I have marked my choice below.

☐ I agree with the $ _____ fee which my representative is asking to charge and collect. By signing this request, I am not giving up my right to disagree later with the total fee amount the Social Security Administration authorizes my representative to charge and collect.

OR

☐ I do not agree with the requested fee or other information given here, or I need more time. I understand I must call, visit, or write to SSA within 20 days if I have questions or if I disagree with the fee requested or any information shown (as explained on the reverse sides of this form).

Signature of Claimant _____ Date _____

Address (include Zip Code) _____ Telephone No. and Area Code _____

Form SSA-1560-U4 (12-89)
Destroy prior editions

FILE COPY

INSTRUCTIONS FOR USING THIS PETITION

Any attorney or other representative who wants to charge or collect a fee for services, rendered in connection with a claim before the Social Security Administration (SSA), is required by law to first obtain SSA's approval of the fee [sections 206 (a) and 1631 (d) (2) of the Social Security Act (42 U.S.C. 406 (a) and 1383 (d) (2)); section 413 (b) of the Black Lung Benefits Act (30 U.S.C. 923 (b)); and sections 404.1720, 410.686b, and 416.1520 of Social Security Administration Regulations Numbers 4, 10, and 16, respectively].

The only exceptions are if the fee is for services rendered (1) when a nonprofit organization or government agency pays the fee and any expenses out of funds which a government entity provided or administered and the claimant incurs no liability, directly or indirectly, for the cost of such services and expenses; (2) in an official capacity such as that of legal guardian, committee, or similar court-appointed office and the court has approved the fee in question; or (3) in representing the claimant before a court of law. A representative who has rendered services in a claim before both SSA and a court of law may seek a fee from either or both, but generally neither tribunal has the authority to set a fee for services rendered before the other [42 U.S.C. 406 (a) and (b)].

When to File a Fee Petition

The representative should request fee approval only after completing all services (for the claimant and any auxiliaries). The representative has the option to petition either before or after SSA effectuates the determination(s).

In order to receive direct payment of all or any part of an authorized fee from past-due benefits, the attorney representative should file a request for fee approval, or written notice of intent to file a request, within 60 days of the date the notice of the favorable determination is mailed. When there are multiple claims on one account and the attorney will not file the petition within 60 days after the mailing date of the first notice of favorable determination, he or she should file a written notice of intent to file a request for fee approval within the 60-day period.

Where to File the Petition

The representative must first give the "Claimant's Copy" of the SSA-1560-U4 petition to the claimant for whom he or she rendered services, with a copy of each attachment. The representative may then file the original and third carbon copy, the "OHA Copy," of the SSA-1560-U4, and the attachment(s), with the appropriate SSA office:

* If a court or the Appeals Council issued the decision, send the petition to the Office of Hearings and Appeals, Attention: Attorney Fee Branch, P.O. Box 3200, Arlington, VA 22203.

* If an Administrative Law Judge issued the decision, send the petition to him or her using the hearing office address.

* In all other cases, send the petition to the reviewing office address which appears at the top right of the notice of award or notice of disapproved claim.

Evaluation of a Petition for a Fee

If the claimant has not agreed to and signed the fee petition, SSA does not begin evaluating the request for 30 days. SSA must decide what is a reasonable fee for the services rendered to the claimant, keeping in mind the purpose of the social security, black lung, or supplemental security income program. When evaluating a request for fee approval, SSA will consider the (1) extent and type of services the representative performed; (2) complexity of the case; (3) level of skill and competence required of the representative in giving the services; (4) amount of time he or she spent on the case; (5) results achieved; (6) levels of review to which the representative took the claim and at which he or she became the representative; and (7) amount of fee requested for services rendered, including any amount authorized or requested before but excluding any amount of expenses incurred.

SSA also considers the amount of benefits payable, if any, but authorizes the fee amount based on consideration of all the factors given here. The amount of benefits payable in a claim is determined by specific provision of law unrelated to the representative's efforts. Also, the amount of past due benefits may depend on the length of time that has elapsed since the claimant's effective date of entitlement.

Disagreement

SSA notifies both the representative and the claimant of the amount which it authorizes the representative to charge. If either or both disagree, SSA will further review the fee authorization when the representative sends a letter, explaining the reason(s) for disagreement, to the appropriate office within 30 days after the date of the notice of authorization to charge and receive a fee.

Collection of the Fee

Basic liability for payment of a representative's approved fee rests with the client. However, SSA will assist in fee collection when the representative is an attorney and SSA awards the claimant benefits under Title II of the Social Security Act or Title IV of the Federal Coal Mine Health and Safety Act of 1969, as amended. In these cases, SSA generally withholds 25 per cent of the claimant's past-due benefits. Once the fee is approved, SSA pays the attorney from the claimant's withheld funds. This does not mean that SSA will approve as a reasonable fee 25 per cent of past due benefits. The amount that is payable to the attorney from the withheld benefits is subject to offset by any fee payment(s) the attorney has received or expects to receive from an escrow or trust account. If the approved fee is more than the amount of the withheld benefits, collection of the difference is a matter between the attorney and the client.

Penalty for Charging or Collecting an Unauthorized Fee

Any individual who charges or collects an unauthorized fee for services provided in any claim, including services before a court which has rendered a favorable determination, may be subject to prosecution under 42 U.S.C. 406 and 1383 which provide that such individual, upon conviction thereof, shall for each offense be punished by a fine not exceeding $500, or by imprisonment not exceeding one year, or both. These penalties do not apply to fees for services performed before a court in supplemental security income claims because section 1383 provides no controls over such fees.

Computer Matching

We may also use the information you give us when we match records by computer. Matching programs compare our records with those of other Federal, State, or local government agencies. Many agencies may use matching programs to find or prove that a person qualifies for benefits paid by the Federal government. The law allows us to do this even if you do not agree to it.

These and other reasons why information about you may be used or given out are explained in the Federal Register. If you want to learn more about this, contact any Social Security office.

Public Reporting Burden

Public reporting burden for this collection of information is estimated to average 30 minutes per response, including the time for reviewing instructions, searching existing data sources, gathering and maintaining the data needed, and completing and reviewing the collection of information. Send comments regarding this burden estimate or any other aspect of this collection of information, including suggestions for reducing this burden, to the Social Security Administration, ATTN: Reports Clearance Officer, 1-A-21 Operations Bldg., Baltimore, MD 21235 and to the Office of Information and Regulatory Affairs, Office of Management and Budget, Washington, DC 20503.

REQUEST FOR REVIEW OF HEARING DECISION/ORDER
(Take or mail original and all copies to your local Social Security office)

See Privacy Act
Notice on Reverse

CLAIMANT	(Check ONE) Initial Entitlement ☐	Termination or other Postentitlement Action ☐

WAGE EARNER (Leave blank if same as above)

Type Claim (Check ONE)

Retirement or Survivors	Only	[ ] (RSI)
Disability, Worker or Child	Only	[ ] (DIWC)
Disability, Widow or Widower	Only	[ ] (DIWW)
Health Insurance, Part A	Only	[ ] (HIA)
SSI, Aged . . . . . . Only [ ] (SSIA) With Title II Claim		[ ] (SSAC)
SSI, Blind . . . . . . Only [ ] (SSIB) With Title II Claim		[ ] (SSBC)
SSI, Disability . . . Only [ ] (SSID) With Title II Claim		[ ] (SSDC)
Other (Specify)		

SOCIAL SECURITY NUMBER

SPOUSE'S NAME AND SOCIAL SECURITY NUMBER
(Complete ONLY in Supplemental Security Income Case)

NAME	SSN

I disagree with the action taken on the above claim and request review of such action by the Appeals Council of the Office of Hearings and Appeals. My reasons for disagreement are:

ADDITIONAL EVIDENCE

Any additional evidence which you wish to submit must be either attached to this form or forwarded within 15 days to the Appeals Council at the address shown below. It is important that you write your Social Security number on any letter or material you send us. Where the evidence is not submitted within 15 days of this date, or within any extension of time granted by the Appeals Council, the Council will proceed to take its action based on the evidence of record.

Knowing that anyone making a false statement or representation of a material fact for use in determining the right to payment under the Social Security Act commits a crime punishable under Federal law, I certify that the above statements are true.

Signed by: (Either the claimant or representatives should sign—Enter addresses for both)

SIGNATURE OR NAME OF CLAIMANT'S REPRESENTATIVE ☐ ATTORNEY ☐ NON ATTORNEY	CLAIMANT SIGNATURE
STREET ADDRESS	STREET ADDRESS
CITY, STATE, AND ZIP CODE	CITY, STATE, AND ZIP CODE
AREA CODE AND TELEPHONE NUMBER	DATE	AREA CODE AND TELEPHONE NUMBER

Claimant should not fill in below this line

TO BE COMPLETED BY SOCIAL SECURITY ADMINISTRATION

Is this request filed timely?   ☐ Yes ☐ No   If "NO" is checked: (1) attach claimant's explanation for delay; (2) attach any pertinent letter, material or information in Social Security Office.

ACKNOWLEDGEMENT OF RECEIPT OF REQUEST FOR REVIEW OF HEARING DECISION/ORDER

This request for Review of Hearing Decision/Order was filed on _____ at _____
The APPEALS COUNCIL will notify you of its action on your request.

	For the Social Security Administration:
	SIGNATURE BY:
	TITLE
	STREET ADDRESS
APPEALS COUNCIL OFFICE OF HEARINGS AND APPEALS, SSA P.O. BOX 3200 ARLINGTON, VA 22203	CITY
	STATE	ZIP CODE
	SERVICING SOCIAL SECURITY OFFICE CODE

PAPERWORK/PRIVACY ACT NOTICE

The Social Security Act (sections 205(a), 702, 1631(e)(1)(A) and (B), and 1869(b)(1) and (c), as appropriate) authorizes the collection of information on this form. We need the information to continue processing your claim. You do not have to give it, but if you do not you may not receive benefits under the Social Security Act. We may give out the information on this form without your written consent if we need to get more information to decide if you are eligible for benefits or if a Federal law requires us to do so. Specifically, we may provide information to another Federal, State, or local government agency which is deciding your eligibility for a government benefit or program; to the President or a Congressman inquiring on your behalf; to an independent party who needs statistical information for a research paper or audit report on a Social Security program; or to the Department of Justice to represent the Federal Government in a court suit related to a program administered by the Social Security Administration. We explain, in the Federal Register, these and other reasons why we may use or give out information about you. If you would like more information, get in touch with any Social Security Office .

Notes

Date:_____

_____
_____
_____
_____

Date:_____

_____
_____
_____
_____

Date:_____

_____
_____
_____

Date:_____

_____
_____
_____

Date:_____

_____
_____
_____
_____

Date:_____

_____
_____
_____
_____

Date:_____

_____
_____
_____
_____

Date:_____

_____
_____
_____

Date:_____

_____
_____
_____
_____

Date:_____

_____
_____
_____
_____

Date:_____

_____
_____
_____
_____

Date:_____

_____
_____
_____

Appendix C

Book Forms

Notes

Date:_____

_____
_____
_____
_____

Date:_____

_____
_____
_____
_____

Date:_____

_____
_____
_____
_____

Date:_____

_____
_____
_____
_____

Chronic Illness Survey

Gathering statistical information is the first step in any project. Please fill in as much as possible. You may add your name if you wish, or just use your initials. At the present time there is no formal research and the statistical information will be shared only with your permission to those who are involved in research or provide Health Care Services.

Today's date_____   Age_____
Age at Diagnosis_____

Male__ Female__ Ancestry background
(Scandinavian, European, etc.)_____

Where did you live when
diagnosed?_____

When did you first notice
symptoms?_____

When did you first seek medical
attention?_____

_____

What are your current
symptoms?_____

_____

_____

How long did it take for a doctor to make a
diagnosis?_____

What was the
diagnosis?_____

How was the diagnosis
made?_____

Who made the diagnosis (GP, Ophthalmologist,
etc.)?_____

What kind of tests have you had?
Results? _____
_____
_____

Have any tests been repeated?
Results?_____
_____

What kind of specialists have you
seen?_____
_____

Have you tried any treatment "outside" traditional
medicine? What? (chiropractic, Herbalists
etc.)_____

How often do you see your regular
doctor?_____   Specialist?_____

Do you use any type of therapy?
(PT, Occupational, Psychological,etc.)_____
_____

What medications do you currently take?
(Rx. OTC, regularly, occasionally)_____
_____

Do you have other health problems?
(Allergy,diabetes,etc.)_____
_____

Do any blood relatives have a chronic illness?_____
The same as you?_____

Please check each condition that applies:
___Alcoholism ___Other substance dependent disorders
___Allergies ___Alzheimers ___Arthritis ___Asthma
___Diabetes ___Heart ___Kidney ___Liver ___Lung
___Lupus___Multiple Sclerosis___Muscular Dystrophy
___Myasthenia Gravis ___Neuropathy ___Osteoporosis
___Parkinson's ___Stroke ___Vision disturbance
Other_____

Have you ever smoked?_____ Do you smoke now?_____
How long?_____ How much? _____

Are you currently working?___

Type of Employment _____

If no: Have you ever worked?___
Type of work_____

Number of hours per day____

Number of hours per week____

Are you working at the same job as when you were
first diagnosed?_____

Have you changed employment because of medical
problems?___ If yes, would you explain?_____

_____

_____

_____

Has your employer/workplace made any changes
to accommodate your needs?_____

How?_____

_____

_____

What coping skills do you use?_____

_____

How has your illness changed your life?_____

_____

What resources do you use? (Networking, books, etc.)

_____

_____

Have you changed your living environment?
(Stairs, walking aids, etc.)_____

_____

Do you have any special needs? (List most troublesome
first)_____

_____

_____

Do you belong to a support group?___

Who sponsors group?_____

How often does it meet?_____

Has it helped you? How/Why_____

_____

_____

Do you keep a health diary so that you can keep your family and physicians aware of your daily and weekly condition? (Some changes are very minute and hard to recognize and or remember)._____

Other comments _____
_____
_____
_____
_____
_____

For statistical studies please give

City_____ State_____ Zip_____

Optional: Name _____

Address_____

Telephone (_ _ _) _ _ _ _ _ _ _

I give PC Publications permission to release information to those involved in research.

_____
Signature

Please mail survey to PC Publications
P. O. Box 1593
Piscataway, N.J. 08855-1593

Help Us Discover More Physicians

Do you know of a Physician Associated with Sarcoidosis not included in this listing?

Physician

_____

_____

Street Address

_____

City_____**State**_____

Zip_____   **Tel. (_ _ _) _ _ _ - _ _ _ _**

Physician

_____

_____

Street Address

_____

City_____**State**_____

Zip_____   **Tel. (_ _ _) _ _ _ - _ _ _ _**

Physician

_____

_____

Street Address

_____

City_____State_____

Zip_____   Tel. (_ _ _) _ _ _ - _ _ _ _

Physician

_____

_____

Street Address

_____

City_____State_____

Zip_____   Tel. (_ _ _) _ _ _ - _ _ _ _

Physician

_____

_____

Street Address

_____

City_____State_____

Zip_____   Tel. (_ _ _) _ _ _ - _ _ _ _

Physician

_____

_____

Street Address

_____

City_____State_____

Zip_____   Tel. (_ _ _) _ _ _ - _ _ _ _

Physician

_____

_____

Street Address

_____

City_____State_____

Zip_____   Tel. (_ _ _) _ _ _ - _ _ _ _

Please Mail Forms To:

PC Publications
P.O. Box 1593
Piscataway, N.J. 08855-1593
Or Call PC Publications at (908) 699-0733

Help Us Discover More

Sarcoidosis Support Groups

Do you know of a group not included in this listing?

Group's
Name_____

Contact Person's
Name_____

Title or Affiliation with the
Group_____

Street
Address_____

(City)_____(State)_____

(Zip)_____

Please Mail This Form To:

PC Publications
P.O. Box 1593
Piscataway, N.J. 08855-1593
Or Call PC Publications at (908) 699-0733

Do you need to make changes in any of the listing?

Group's
Name_____

Contact Person's
Name_____

Title or Affiliation with the
Group_____

Street
Address_____

(City)_____(State)_____

(Zip) _____

Phone
Number_____

Please Mail This Form To:

PC Publications
P.O. Box 1593
Piscataway, N.J. 08855-1593
Or Call PC Publications at (908) 699-0733

ORDER FORM

For additional copies of the Sarcoidosis Resource Guide and Directory, please use this order form,

Mail orders to:

PC Publications, P.O. Box 1593
Piscataway, N.J. 08855-1593
or you may call (908) 699-0733

Quantity	Item	Price	Amount
	Sarcoidosis Resource Guide and Directory	**19.95**	
			Sub total
			Tax (7%)*
			Postage**
			Total

(Please make checks payable to PC Publications)

NAME_____

ADDRESS_____

CITY_____STATE_____ ZIP_____

Should we need to contact you about your order, please provide your telephone number: (_____) - _____ - _____

*New Jersey State residents only.
**Postage and Handling: $2.00 for first book and $1.00 for each additional book.
Please allow 6-8 weeks for delivery.

INDEX

A

Administrative Law Judge (ALJ) 82, 83, 84, 85, 86
AIDS 29, 113
Alabama, University Of 131
Alexander-Thomas, Dr. Nanette 35, 148
Allegheny General Hospital 45
Alliance for Disabled in Action 178
Alveolitis 21
American Lung Association 173
Anemia 16
Angina Pectoris 16
Arnet, Dr. Frank 155
Ausley, Geneva 179
Arthritis, Migratory 36
Austin, Dr. Joseph 148

B

Baum, Dr. G. 43
BCG Vaccination 219
Besnier, Ernest 215
Beth Israel Medical Center 144
Bielory, Dr. Leonard 145, 197
Blackman, Dr. Francis 146
Blau 38
Blau's Syndrome 38
Blau, Dr. E. 42
Boeck, Dr. Caesar 15, 216

K

L

O

P